Clinical Management of Fibromyalgia

First Edition

Don L. Goldenberg, MD
Professor of Medicine
Tufts University School of Medicine

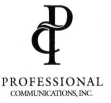

PROFESSIONAL
COMMUNICATIONS, INC.

Professional Communications, Inc.
A Medical Publishing Company

Marketing Office:
400 Center Bay Drive
West Islip, NY 11795
(t) 631/661-2852
(f) 631/661-2167

Editorial Office:
PO Box 10
Caddo, OK 74729-0010
(t) 580/367-9838
(f) 580/367-9989

For orders only, please call
1-800-337-9838
or visit our website at
www.pcibooks.com

ISBN: 978-1-932610-40-6

Printed in the United States of America

DISCLAIMER
The opinions expressed in this publication reflect those of the author. However, the author makes no warranty regarding the contents of the publication. The protocols described herein are general and may not apply to a specific patient. Any product mentioned in this publication should be taken in accordance with the prescribing information provided by the manufacturer.

This text is printed on recycled paper.

TABLE OF CONTENTS

TABLES

FIGURES

1

What Is Fibromyalgia?

Fibromyalgia (FM) is a chronic pain disorder characterized by:
- Widespread muscle pain
- Tender soft-tissue spots throughout the body
- Systemic complaints, including:
  - Fatigue
  - Sleep disturbances
  - Mood disturbances
  - Headaches
  - Bowel irritability.

FM is found worldwide, with an estimated prevalence of 1% to 4% of the general population.[1] In rheumatology clinics, 70% to 90% of patients have been female but in population-based studies, the female-to-male ratio has been 3 to 1.[2] The typical age at onset is 35 to 55 years, with prevalence of FM increasing with age, reaching 7% to 8% in women of age 60 to 80 years. FM occurs with similar frequency in children and adolescents, although only a few epidemiologic studies in children have been reported. The clinical manifestations of FM in children have been very similar to those in adults.

Most often, FM occurs in otherwise healthy individuals (**Table 1.1**). About 50% of FM patients do not recall any precipitating factors at the onset of their symptoms. Many recall having aches and pains and fatigue since early childhood. The other 50% of FM patients attribute the onset of their condition to a specific event, including physical or emotional trauma or an infection. FM may develop following Lyme disease, even after appropriate antibiotic treatment eradicates the infection. Patients may be then inappropriately diagnosed with chronic Lyme disease and treated with repeated courses of antibiotics to no avail. Nonspecific viral infections are the most common precipitating factors in some studies of FM. Most often, the presumed inciting factor does not appear to change the course of a patient's FM. One exception may be so-

TABLE 1.1 — Who Gets Fibromyalgia?

- No concurrent medical illness:
  - Any age, but peak age 40 to 60 years
  - 60% to 90% female in clinic, but less in population
- Concurrent medical illness (eg, SLE, RA, OA, hypothyroidism, hepatitis); important to consider in patients with rheumatic or chronic pain disorders
- Prior medical illness (eg, Lyme disease, viral illness)
- Medications (steroid taper)

called posttraumatic FM. Patients who attribute the onset of FM to events (eg, motor vehicle accidents or trauma at work) have, in general, poorer outcomes. They may more often be involved in litigation and disability issues.

FM also may coexist with systemic diseases such as rheumatoid arthritis (RA), systemic lupus erythematosus (SLE), or hypothyroidism (**Table 1.1**). The prevalence of FM in SLE has varied from 15% to 40%.[3] There is also an increased prevalence of FM in RA, osteoarthritis (OA), and Sjögren's syndrome. In patients with RA, the presence of FM is associated with more pain and a poorer outcome.[4] Some studies report that FM is more common in patients with hepatitis, hypothyroidism, and other systemic diseases. Certain medications, notably steroid withdrawal, may also trigger FM.

Although there are no definitive findings on physical examination and in laboratory testing, the diagnosis of FM should be fairly straightforward. Nevertheless, the recognition of FM as a specific illness is complicated by the lack of objective (or structural) abnormalities. FM should be strongly considered when a patient complains of aches and pain for months but the physical examination is normal, or the patient reports numbness, tingling, and burning, but the neurologic examination is also normal.

Most patients also have multiple other, unexplained somatic symptoms and the initial workup includes a normal complete blood count (CBC), erythrocyte sedimentation rate (ESR), and thyroid function tests.

FM is often classified as a functional illness, as are common disorders often comorbid with FM, including:

- Chronic low back pain
- Chronic headaches
- Irritable bowel syndrome (IBS)
- Chronic fatigue syndrome (CFS)
- Temporomandibular joint (TMJ) pain
- Vulvodynia
- Interstitial cystitis or irritable bladder syndrome
- Mood disturbances.

These disorders are characterized by organ dysfunction rather than organ damage, the most consistent being abnormal pain processing in the central nervous system (CNS).

Historical Perspective

References to FM date back to antiquity and are found throughout the Bible[5]:

> ... and wearisome nights are appointed to me. When I lie down, I say, When I shall arise, and the night be gone? Am I full of tossings and turnings to and fro from unto the dawning of the day (Job 7:3-4), ... and the days of affliction have taken hold of me. My bones are pierced in the night and my sinews take no rest (Job 30:16-17).

The overlap of chronic fatigue and chronic pain was suggested in 1750 by Sir Richard Manningham, under the term "febricula," described as *listlessness, with great lassitude and weariness all over the body...little frying pans...the patient is a little...forgetful.*[6] The current designation of FM and CFS in the 19th century were often called neurasthenia or myalgic encephalitis.

FM was initially termed fibrositis by Sir William Gowers, a neurologist, in 1904 (**Figure 1.1**).[7] A pathologist in Glasgow, Ralph Stockman, demonstrated inflammatory muscle changes in fibrositis, but during the next century, most investigators could not confirm that

FIGURE 1.1 — Initial Description of Fibromyalgia

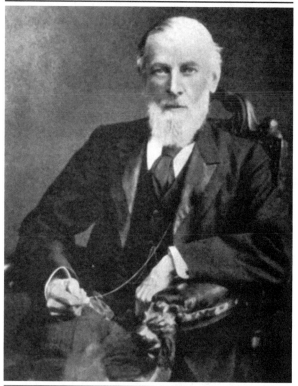

- Descriptions of musculoskeletal aches and pains date to the late 16th century: "rheumatism"
- Sir William Gowers:
  - British neurologist who coined the term fibrositis in 1904
  - Defining his own low back pain as a form of muscular rheumatism
- Various historical explanations:
  - Infection
  - Inflammation of fibrous muscle tissue
  - Edematous fat lobules

tissue inflammation was present. In the 1930s, Lewis and Kellgren demonstrated that muscle pain was often referred away from the initial site of noxious stimuli and this referral pattern was not dermatomal in nature. Although subtle electron microscopic muscle abnormalities were reported, when studies controlled for activity and exercise, no significant pathology was found. The absence of tissue inflammation led some to conclude that FM should be called psychogenic rheumatism. Many examples of FM have been depicted in the Arts, none more striking than Frida Kahlo's self-portrait in 1916, following a life of chronic pain after her tragic bus accident (**Figure 1.2**).[8]

The current concept that FM is a disorder of the central nervous system followed Moldofsky's recognition of sleep abnormalities in FM in 1975.[9] In 1981, Yunus and others characterized the major clinical signs and symptoms and suggested diagnostic criteria for FM.[10] In 1990, the American College of Rheumatology (ACR) FM classification criteria were published, ushering in the modern concept of FM and the >3000 peer-reviewed studies on FM during the past 20 years.[11]

FIGURE 1.2 — Frida Kahlo Self Portrait, 1916

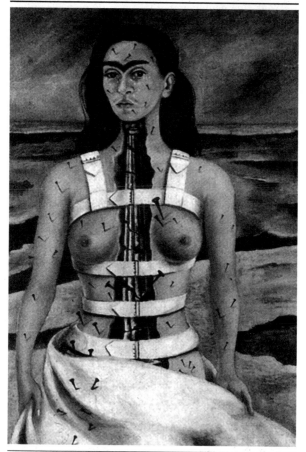

Self-portrait by Frida Kahlo may represent her battle with symptoms of fibromyalgia after a serious accident.

Martinez-Lavin M, et al. *Arthritis Rheum*. 2000;43(3):708-709.

REFERENCES

1. Wolfe F, Ross K, Anderson J, Russell IJ, Hebert L. The prevalence and characteristics of fibromyalgia in the general population. *Arthritis Rheum.* 1995;38(1):19-28.

2. Croft P, Rigby AS, Boswell R, Schollum J, Silman A. The prevalence of chronic widespread pain in the general population. *J Rheumatol.* 1993;20(4):710-713.

3. Middleton GD, McFarlin JE, Lipsky PE. The prevalence and clinical impact of fibromyalgia in systemic lupus erythematosus. *Arthritis Rheum.* 1994;37(8):1181-1188.

4. Wolfe F, Michaud K. Severe rheumatoid arthritis (RA), worse outcomes, comorbid illness, and sociodemographic disadvantage characterize RA patients with fibromyalgia. *J Rheumatol.* 2004;31(4):695-700.

5. Wallace DJ. Fibromyalgia: unusual historical aspects and new pathogenic insights. *Mt Sinai J Med.* 1984;51(2):124-131.

6. Sharpe M. Chronic fatigue syndrome. *Psychiatr Clin North Am.* 1996;19(3):549-573.

7. Gowers WR. Lumbago: its lessons and analogues. *Br Med.* 1904;1:117-121.

8. Martínez-Lavín M, Amigo MC, Coindreau J, Canoso J. Fibromyalgia in Frida Kahlo's life and art. *Arthritis Rheum.* 2000;43(3):708-709.

9. Moldofsky H. Sleep and fibrositis syndrome. *Rheum Dis Clin North Am.* 1989;15(1):91-103.

10. Yunus M, Masi AT, Calabro JJ, Miller KA, Feigenbaum SL. Primary fibromyalgia (fibrositis): clinical study of 50 patients with matched normal controls. *Semin Arthritis Rheum.* 1981;11(1):151-171.

11. Wolfe F, Smythe HA, Yunus MB, et al. The American College of Rheumatology 1990 Criteria for the Classification of Fibromyalgia. Report of the Multicenter Criteria Committee. *Arthritis Rheum.* 1990;33(2):160-172.

2

Diagnosis and Differential Diagnosis

Diagnosis

The cardinal symptoms of FM, widespread pain and fatigue, are initial symptoms in a multitude of illnesses, including common occurrences such as the flu or overexertion. Therefore, the diagnosis of FM should not be seriously considered until these complaints have been persistent for at least 3 months. At that point, a careful patient history and examination are the only tools necessary to make the diagnosis.[1]

The initial patient evaluation should begin with a thorough review of the available clinical records. The patient should be asked how the symptoms began, how they impact on their life and work, what aggravates the symptoms, and what makes them better. Inquiring about mood, stress, and sleep is essential. When appropriate, a more detailed sleep questionnaire, a psychiatric history, and mental status examination should be performed. Activity and exercise levels should be assessed. All current and prior medications must be documented, including alternative and nonprescription items. A standardized FM form can be used to streamline documentation.

The pain of FM is, by definition, widespread, involving both sides of the body and above and below the waist. Although many descriptions have been used by patients in their reporting of the pain, telltale symptoms include "I feel as if I hurt all over" or "it feels as if I always have the flu" (**Table 2.1**). Patients typically describe that the pain is predominantly throughout the muscles but sometimes they will also state that their joints hurt and sometimes describe swelling in the joints. However, in FM, unless there is concurrent arthritis, such as RA or OA, joint swelling does not occur. FM patients also report paresthesias, including numbness, tingling, burning, creeping, or crawling sensations, especially in both arms and both legs. However, unless a concurrent neurologic disorder

TABLE 2.1 — Telltale Patient Descriptions of Fibromyalgia

- "I feel as if I hurt all over!"
- "It feels as if I always have the flu!"
- "No matter how much sleep I get, it feels like a truck ran me over when I get up!"

(eg, carpal tunnel syndrome or a cervical radiculopathy) is present, a detailed neurologic evaluation or formal testing is unremarkable.

The other universal symptom of FM is fatigue. This is especially notable when arising from sleep but also is prominent in the mid afternoon. Seemingly minor activities aggravate the pain and fatigue, although prolonged inactivity also heightens these symptoms. Patients are stiff in the morning and feel unrefreshed, even if they have slept 8 to 10 hours. FM patients characteristically sleep lightly, waking frequently during early morning and having difficulty getting back to sleep. A common quote is "No matter how much sleep I get, it feels like a truck ran me over in the morning." Headaches are present in >50% of FM patients and include migraine and muscular (tension) types. Cognitive disturbances and mood disturbances are also present in the majority of patients.[2]

In patients with FM, the only reproducible finding on physical examination is tenderness in specific anatomic locations, termed "tender points." In 1990, the ACR Classification Criteria for Fibromyalgia was published, using the tender-point examination as part of the diagnostic criteria.[3] The classification criteria were established after a number of rheumatologists determined the optimal historical and physical findings that could differentiate patients with FM from those with other rheumatic diseases and other forms of chronic pain. These criteria were then field tested in a number of academic rheumatology clinics and office practices. The criteria included the symptom of widespread pain, including above and below the waist as well as the right and left sides of the body, and the physical finding of at least 11 of 18 tender points (**Figure 2.1**). These simple criteria provided >85% specificity and sensitivity in differentiating patients with FM from those with other rheumatic diseases.

FIGURE 2.1 — American College of Rheumatology Diagnostic Criteria for Fibromyalgia

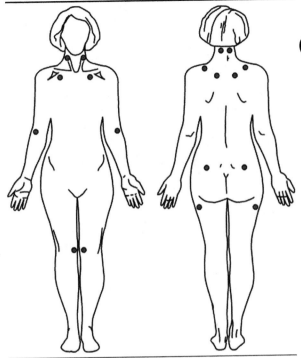

- ACR diagnostic criteria:
  - Both sensitive (88.4%) and specific (81.1%)
  - History of CWP ≥3 months
  - Patients must exhibit ≥11 of 18 tender points
- FM can be identified from among other rheumatologic conditions with use of ACR criteria

The tender-point examination requires that the examiner knows where to palpate and how much pressure to apply (**Figure 2.2**). The nine pair of tender points used for the ACR Criteria are found at locations that most primary care physicians and specialists routinely evaluate in patients with soft-tissue complaints. These locations include:

- Upper mid trapezius muscle
- Lateral epicondyle (the so-called tennis elbow location)

FIGURE 2.2 — The Tender-Point Examination

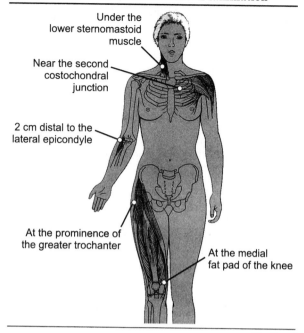

Under the lower sternomastoid muscle

Near the second costochondral junction

2 cm distal to the lateral epicondyle

At the prominence of the greater trochanter

At the medial fat pad of the knee

Continued

- Second costochondral junction (the site of costochondritis)
- Greater trochanter (the site of trochanteric bursitis of the hip).

The amount of pressure should equal 4 kg/cm², which is enough to whiten the nail bed of the examiner's finger tip. In research studies, a pressure gauge called a dolorimeter may provide more accuracy, but in the clinic, the examiner's finger will suffice. While evaluating the tenderness of the nine pair of specific FM points, it is recommended that so-called control locations, such as over the thumb, the mid forearm, or the forehead, be palpated in the same fashion. FM patients are typically not as tender in these control areas. However, the FM patient will be more tender in control locations compared with a healthy control subject. A specific joint examination should be

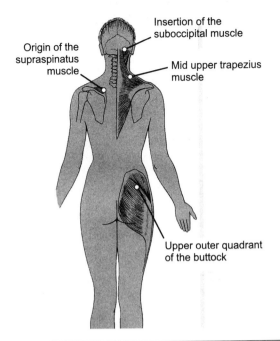

Insertion of the
suboccipital muscle

Origin of the
supraspinatus
muscle

Mid upper trapezius
muscle

Upper outer quadrant
of the buttock

2

1. Use pressure of 4 kg/cm^2 or enough to whiten examiner's fingernail.
2. Apply pressure gradually.
3. Use your finger or thumb.
4. End point is pain.
5. Compare with joint tenderness and always check for joint inflammation.
6. Evaluate control locations.

carried out, looking for any synovitis and also palpating for tenderness over the joints themselves.

The tender points represent heightened pain perception rather than sites of inflammation or tissue pathology. Therefore they are proxies for pain and the exact number necessary to diagnose FM is somewhat arbitrary.[4] It must be remembered that the classification criteria were validated for large patient populations and should be used primarily in clinical research and epidemiologic studies of FM. In the clinic, a patient could be considered to have FM even if the 11 of 18 tender points are not present, provided the history is consistent and the major differential diagnoses have been excluded.

Some investigators have advocated not using the tender-point examination as part of the FM diagnostic criteria. Wolfe, Katz, and colleagues found that the symptom of widespread pain and a patient-completed pain diagram performed as well as the ACR classification criteria (**Figure 2.3**).[5,6] They also found that the presence of six tender points may correlate better with a clinical diagnosis of FM. Hudson and Pope suggested using only symptom criteria, such as the way *Diagnostic and Statistical Manual of Mental Disorders* (*DSM-IV*) criteria for major depressive disorder were validated (**Table 2.2**).[7] In patients with chronic, widespread pain, four of six of the following symptoms were sufficient for the FM diagnosis:

- Generalized fatigue
- Headaches
- Sleep disturbance
- Neuropsychiatric complaints
- Numbness or tingling sensations
- Irritable bowel.

However, performing a tender-point and joint examination should be confirmatory in any patient suspected of having FM.

The initial evaluation of a patient with FM should include some measure of symptom severity (**Figure 2.4**). These forms, such as a 10-cm visual analogue scale, can be completed by the patient, with the patient rating the severity of their primary symptoms, such as pain or fatigue.[8] Such validated instruments can be followed over time to evaluate therapy.

The large number of associated symptoms in FM can be daunting to the clinician. Patients universally complain of exhaustion and nonrestorative sleep (**Figure 2.5**). Many patients with FM describe cognitive issues, especially regarding short-term memory. Facial pain and jaw pain, often associated with dizziness or other vestibular complaints, frequently result in neurologic evaluations. Oral specialists may diagnose TMJ syndrome. Dryness in the eyes and mouth may raise the possibility of Sjögren's

FIGURE 2.3 — Pain Diagram From a Patient With Fibromyalgia

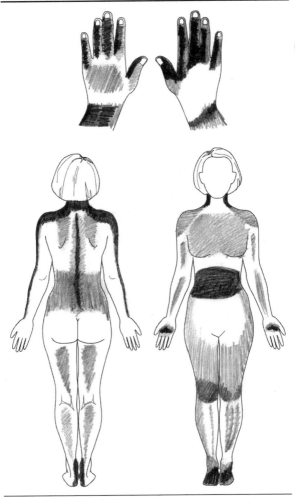

Figure displays pain in all sites as well as intensity of pain as represented by darkness of penciled-in areas.

Wolfe P. *J Rheumatol.* 2003;30(2):369-378.

TABLE 2.2 — Structured Interview for Fibromyalgia

- Generalized, chronic pain (≥3 months) affecting the axial, plus upper and lower segments, plus left and right sides of the body
- At least four of the following symptoms:
  - Generalized fatigue
  - Headaches
  - Sleep disturbance
  - Neuropsychiatric complaints
  - Numbness and/or tingling sensations
  - Irritable bowel symptoms

Pope HG Jr, Hudson JI. *Int J Psychiatry Med*. 1991;21:205-232.

FIGURE 2.4 — Fibromyalgia Symptom Evaluation

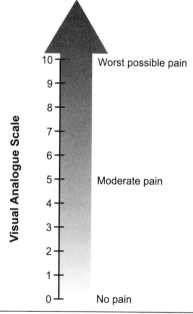

- Symptom activity, severity best measured by self-administered VAS for pain, fatigue, global, mood
- Outcome best evaluated by FIQ or other composite functional scales

FIGURE 2.5 — Fibromyalgia: A Constellation of Symptoms

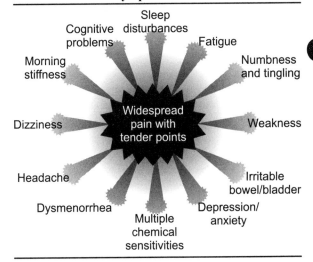

syndrome. FM patients frequently complain of bowel and bladder as well pelvic pain, and may be diagnosed to have interstitial cystitis, IBS, female urethral syndrome, vulvodynia, and vulvar vestibulitis. FM patients report many allergies and medication reactions and are sometimes diagnosed with multiple chemical sensitivity.

The diagnostic evaluation always must be individualized (**Figure 2.6**) and will be very operator dependent.[9] If the physician feels comfortable performing a thorough musculoskeletal and neurologic examination, early referral to a rheumatologist or neurologist may not be necessary. Every FM patient should be evaluated for concurrent mood and sleep disturbances. Many primary care physicians are quite skilled in screening for such disturbances, whereas others may prefer specialty consultation.

Differential Diagnosis

The differential diagnosis of FM at first may appear overwhelming but is really quite straightforward. Rheumatic diseases, including polymyalgia rheumatica

FIGURE 2.6 — Diagnostic Work-Up for Fibromyalgia

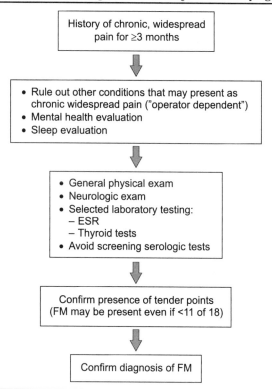

History of chronic, widespread pain for ≥3 months

- Rule out other conditions that may present as chronic widespread pain ("operator dependent")
- Mental health evaluation
- Sleep evaluation

- General physical exam
- Neurologic exam
- Selected laboratory testing:
  - ESR
  - Thyroid tests
- Avoid screening serologic tests

Confirm presence of tender points (FM may be present even if <11 of 18)

Confirm diagnosis of FM

Burckhardt C, et al. Glenview, IL: American Pain Society; 2005. APS Clinical Practice Guidelines Series, No. 4.

(PMR), RA, SLE, and Sjögren's syndrome, may present initially as diffuse pain and fatigue (**Table 2.3**). PMR may mimic FM since there may be no obvious physical findings and patients with both conditions report morning stiffness and fatigue. PMR usually begins after age 60, and often is associated with fever, weight loss, and other systemic signs. In contrast to FM, the ESR is almost always very elevated and patients respond extremely well to modest doses of corticosteroids. The small-joint swelling in the hands and feet characteristic of RA are never part of FM. None of the dermatologic, renal, cardiac,

TABLE 2.3 — Common Conditions Included in Differential Diagnosis of Fibromyalgia

Condition	Distinguishing Features From FM
RA	Joint swelling, deformities, elevated ESR, CRP
SLE	Rash, multisystemic inflammation, very elevated ESR, ANA
PMR	$\geq$60 years of age, severe stiffness, elevated ESR
Myositis, myopathies	Weakness, elevated muscle enzymes
Ankylosing spondylitis	Back, neck immobility, elevated ESR, x-ray changes
Hypothyroidism	Abnormal thyroid function tests
Neuropathies	Weakness, loss of sensation, abnormal EMG, NCV

or other systemic manifestations of SLE or Sjögren's syndrome are found in FM.

Ankylosing spondylitis or other inflammatory back conditions may mimic FM when patients present with axial skeleton pain and stiffness, but the characteristic radiologic features of spondylitis are diagnostic. Inflammatory myositis and metabolic myopathies cause muscle weakness and muscle fatigue but usually are not associated with diffuse pain. Furthermore, patients with FM do not have significant muscle weakness, other than that related to pain or disuse, and they have normal muscle enzyme tests and normal or nonspecific histopathologic findings on muscle biopsy. A fishing expedition for a systemic connective tissue disease is likely to be misleading. The only routine test recommended is an ESR or a C-reactive protein (CRP), as well as a CBC (**Table 2.4**). Since FM is not an inflammatory condition, normal acute-phase reactants immediately provide confidence that an occult inflammatory disorder is unlikely. Serologic tests (eg, antinuclear antibody [ANA] and rheumatoid factor) should only be ordered when the history and examination point to an inflammatory systemic disease. They are often positive in otherwise healthy people.

Endocrine disorders that cause unexplained fatigue and muscles aches, most notably hypothyroidism, may

TABLE 2.4 — Laboratory Evaluation in Fibromyalgia

- In most patients:
  - ESR or CRP
  - CBC
  - Thyroid function tests
- In some patients:
  - Liver function tests
  - CPK
- Avoid serologic screening tests, such as:
  - ANA
  - Rheumatoid factor unless clinical suspicion of systemic connective tissue disease
- Avoid extensive neurologic testing, x-rays, or imaging unless clinical picture warrants

---

mimic FM. It is reasonable to obtain thyroid function tests routinely in the work-up for possible FM. Since FM patients often complain of headaches and paresthesias, peripheral neuropathies, entrapment syndromes (such as carpal tunnel syndrome), and neurologic disorders (such as multiple sclerosis and myasthenia gravis) are sometimes considered in the differential diagnosis. Nonicteric hepatitis may present as exhaustion and myalgias. It is reasonable to have thyroid function and liver function tests done, plus a creatine phosphokinase (CPK), during the initial evaluation. Tests such as an electromyography (EMG) and nerve conduction velocities, should be limited to patients with abnormal neurologic findings (**Table 2.4**).

Since FM can complicate rheumatic and systemic diseases, it is more difficult to diagnose FM in patients with those conditions. For example, a patient who complains of exhaustion, generalized achiness, muscle soreness, and morning stiffness but whose RA is in remission should be evaluated for FM rather than just assuming that the RA is active. This situation warrants early referral to a rheumatologist.

REFERENCES

1. Goldenberg DL. Fibromyalgia syndrome a decade later: what have we learned? *Arch Intern Med*. 1999;159(8):777-785.

2. Glass JM, Park DC, Minear M, Crofford LJ. Memory beliefs and function in fibromyalgia patients. *J Psychosom Res*. 2005;58(3):263-269.

3. Wolfe F, Smythe HA, Yunus MB, et al. The American College of Rheumatology 1990 Criteria for the Classification of Fibromyalgia. Report of the Multicenter Criteria Committee. *Arthritis Rheum*. 1990;33(2):160-172.

4. Wolfe F. The relation between tender points and fibromyalgia symptom variables: evidence that fibromyalgia is not a discrete disorder in the clinic. *Ann Rheum Dis*. 1997;56(4):268-271.

5. Wolfe F. Pain extent and diagnosis: development and validation of the regional pain scale in 12,799 patients with rheumatic disease. *J Rheumatol*. 2003;30(2):369-378.

6. Katz RS, Wolfe F, Michaud K. Fibromyalgia diagnosis: a comparison of clinical, survey, and American College of Rheumatology criteria. *Arthritis Rheum*. 2006;54(1):169-176.

7. Hudson JI, Pope HG. The concept of affective spectrum disorder: relationship to fibromyalgia and other syndromes of chronic fatigue and chronic muscle pain. *Baillieres Clin Rheumatol*. 1994;8(4):839-856.

8. Wolfe F, Ross K, Anderson J, Russell IJ, Hebert L. The prevalence and characteristics of fibromyalgia in the general population. *Arthritis Rheum*. 1995;38(1):19-28.

9. Goldenberg DL, Burckhardt C, Crofford L. Management of fibromyalgia syndrome. *JAMA*. 2004;292(19):2388-2395.

3

Associated Illnesses

The conditions that most often are comorbid with FM include medically unexplained illnesses, such as (**Table 3**.1):

- CFS
- Chronic headache disorders
- IBS
- Irritable bladder or interstitial cystitis
- Vulvodynia
- TMJ pain.

Whether such disorders should be lumped together with FM as multisymptom somatic illnesses or viewed individually is unclear. As with FM, these conditions are diagnosed based on symptoms alone, and not on physical findings or laboratory tests. There is a significant female predominance in these disorders. Each of these conditions is associated with an increased prevalence of mood disorders.

Various subspecialty groups have put forth operational diagnostic criteria for each of these illnesses. For example, CFS is diagnosed only after debilitating fatigue persists or relapses for >6 months and medical or psychiatric disorders that cause chronic fatigue have been excluded.[1] Patients diagnosed with CFS must also have four or more of the following: muscle pain, multijoint pain, impaired memory or concentration, new headaches, nonrestorative sleep, postexertion malaise, sore throat, or tender lymph nodes in the neck or arm. FM has been found in 21% to 80% of CFS patients.[2] The broad range of this association is attributable to differences in definitions of the syndromes and different patient populations studied.

The differential diagnosis of chronic fatigue is broad. Most individuals who have chronic fatigue—and there are 15 million office visits for fatigue each year in the United States—do not have CFS (**Figure 3**.1). Fatigue may be caused by medical diseases such as thyroid deficiency,

TABLE 3.1 — Medically Unexplained Illnesses[a] Concurrent With Fibromyalgia

- CFS
- IBS
- Muscle, migraine headaches
- Irritable bladder syndrome
- Mood disturbances
- Vulvodynia
- TMJ disorder

[a] In each disorder, diagnosis is dependent upon exclusion of disease, symptoms rather than signs, and no reproducible laboratory findings; the gold standard is expert opinion.

FIGURE 3.1 — Chronic Fatigue in the General Population

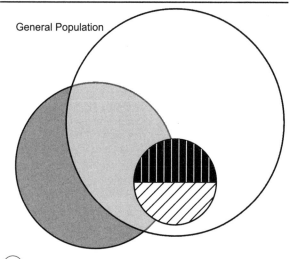

◯ Population affected by prolonged fatigue (≥1 month)

⬤ Overlapping disorder(s) (eg, depression, FM, etc)

▨ CFS: clinically evaluated, unexplained idiopathic chronic fatigue

A conceptual framework of abnormally fatigued populations, including those with CFS and overlapping disorders.

Fukuda K, et al. *Ann Intern Med*. 1994;121:953-959.

anemia, arthritis, or psychiatric disorders, especially depression. The medical nomenclature for chronic idiopathic fatigue has included neurasthenia, benign myalgic encephalomyelitis, and for the past few decades, CFS.

Like FM, CFS is not new. What we now call CFS was described in 1750 by Sir Richard Manningham as "profound listlessness, with great lassitude and weariness all over the body and little flying pains."[3] The American neurologist Dr. George Beard chose the name neurasthenia in 1869 since he believed that the illness was caused by a "weakness of the nerves and nervous exhaustion."[4]

During most of the 20th century, physicians debated whether CFS was an infectious disease. Clusters of cases of what we now call CFS were described in the 1930s through the 1950s throughout the world. In 1934, an outbreak of an illness identical to the current descriptions of CFS occurred in health care workers at Los Angeles County General Hospital. Then in 1984, an epidemic of unexplained fatigue, called a "mysterious, new disease" was reported among residents of Incline Village, Nevada. Most people also had a variety of symptoms that included muscle aches, headaches, diarrhea, dizziness, numbness, tingling, and weakness. Elevated antibody levels to the Epstein-Barr virus were found in these patients with CFS. However, the specificity of these elevated antibody levels to the Epstein-Barr virus was questioned and a team of epidemiologists from the Centers for Disease Control (CDC) found no evidence that this new illness was a specific disease.

Recent recommendations for the evaluation of possible CFS are structured much like those for FM (**Figure 3.2**).[5] Other potential medical and psychiatric causes of chronic fatigue must first be excluded and then patients should meet operational diagnostic criteria based primarily on their symptoms. In addition to the cardinal feature of debilitating chronic fatigue, patients should have four of the following symptoms for 6 months: impaired memory or concentration, sore throat, tender cervical or axillary lymph nodes, muscle pain, multijoint pain, new headaches, unrefreshing sleep, and postexertion malaise. In one report from a CFS clinic, 70% of patients with CFS met criteria for FM.[6]

FIGURE 3.2 — Recommendations for the Evaluation and Classification of Unexplained Chronic Fatigue

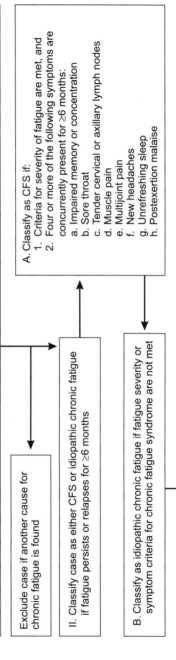

I. Clinically evaluate cases of prolonged or chronic fatigue by:
A. History and physical examination
B. Mental status examination (abnormalities require appropriate psychiatric, psychologic, or neurologic examination)
C. Tests (abnormal results that strongly suggest an exclusionary condition must be resolved):
1. Screening lab tests: CBC, ESR, ALT, total protein, albumin, globulin, alkaline phosphatase, Ca, PO₄, glucose, BUN, electrolytes, creatinine, TSH, and UA
2. Additional tests as clinically indicated to exclude other diagnoses

Exclude case if another cause for chronic fatigue is found

II. Classify case as either CFS or idiopathic chronic fatigue if fatigue persists or relapses for ≥6 months

A. Classify as CFS if:
1. Criteria for severity of fatigue are met, and
2. Four or more of the following symptoms are concurrently present for ≥6 months:
a. Impaired memory or concentration
b. Sore throat
c. Tender cervical or axillary lymph nodes
d. Muscle pain
e. Multijoint pain
f. New headaches
g. Unrefreshing sleep
h. Postexertion malaise

B. Classify as idiopathic chronic fatigue if fatigue severity or symptom criteria for chronic fatigue syndrome are not met

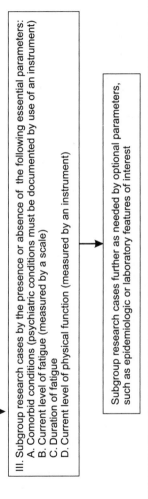

III. Subgroup research cases by the presence or absence of the following essential parameters:
  A. Comorbid conditions (psychiatric conditions must be documented by use of an instrument)
  B. Current level of fatigue (measured by a scale)
  C. Duration of fatigue
  D. Current level of physical function (measured by an instrument)

Subgroup research cases further as needed by optional parameters, such as epidemiologic or laboratory features of interest

Adapted from: Fukuda K, et al. *Ann Intern Med.* 1994;121:953-959.

IBS has been present in 32% to 80% of FM patients (**Table 3.2**). IBS is diagnosed when patients report at least 12 weeks (which need not be consecutive) in the preceding 12 months of abdominal discomfort or pain that has two of the following three features: (1) relief with defecation, (2) onset associated with a change in the frequency of stool (abnormal frequency is >3 times per day or <3 times per week), and (3) onset associated with a change in form (ie, appearance of the stool, where abnormal stool is lumpy/hard or loose/watery).[7]

TABLE 3.2 — Functional Disorders That Often Overlap With Fibromyalgia

Disorder	Overlap (%)
FM and CFS	35-70
FM and IBS	32-80
FM and MCS	33-55
FM and TMD	30-67

Aaron LA, et al. *Arch Intern Med.* 2000;160:221-227.

The prevalence of IBS and depression with FM has varied somewhat with the case definition of IBS. Using the Rome I criteria, the prevalence of IBS was 63% in 105 FM patients, whereas the prevalence increased to 81% utilizing Rome II criteria.[8] These prevalences were much greater in FM patients than in healthy controls. Depression was present in 40% of FM patients compared with 8% of controls. The coexistence of IBS and depression was 31% using Rome I criteria and 34% using the Rome II criteria.

Patients with FM often report sensitivity to various drugs and environmental stimuli. Many meet the criteria for the diagnosis of multiple chemical sensitivity (MCS) syndrome.[9] A 1999 consensus conference on MCS suggested criteria for that diagnosis based on multiple symptoms present in multiple organs occurring on exposure to unrelated chemicals.[10] However, the epidemiologic basis for these diagnostic criteria, as well as the clinical validity of MCS, is very controversial. Nevertheless, 33% to 55% of FM patients do meet criteria for that syndrome (**Table 3.2**).

Musculoskeletal headaches are found in at least 70% of patients with FM and migraine headaches in 30% to 50% of patients.[8] The 1988 International Headache Society Criteria suggest that there should be at least five recurrent headaches lasting for >30 minutes in the past 6 months to diagnose migraine headaches and >10 for tension-type headaches.[10]

3

Many individuals with musculoskeletal headaches also complain of localized neck and shoulder pain, often diagnosed as myofascial pain syndrome. There has been debate whether myofascial pain is merely a localized form of FM or a totally different disorder (**Table 3.3**).

TABLE 3.3 — Myofascial Pain vs Fibromyalgia

Myofascial Pain	Fibromyalgia
• Localized pain	• Widespread pain
• Trigger points	• Tender points
• Taut band	• No muscle pathology
• Specified referral of pain	• Significant mood and sleep disturbances
• Responds to injections	• Poor prognosis
• No significant mood disturbances	
• Good prognosis	

The term myofascial pain has generally been reserved for individuals with muscle pain and trigger points localized to one region of the body, often the head and neck. In contrast, FM is defined by widespread muscle pain. Some investigators believe strongly that electromyographic changes are present in the muscle in myofascial pain and that trigger points can be distinguished from tender points. The trigger point is said to refer pain to a specific anatomic zone and is manifest by a taut band brought out by a snapping sensation to the muscle fibers.[11] The trigger point is also said to refer pain to surrounding tissues in very specific patterns. Trigger points are reported to respond better to injections and manual therapies. There has also been limited evidence that patients with myofascial pain may have fewer mood and sleep disturbances and a better prognosis than those with FM. However, the very few studies to compare FM and myofascial pain found that there was tremendous overlap.[12] Furthermore, FM usually begins in a localized fashion and within months becomes very generalized.

TMJ (temporomandibular joint) syndrome, also called TMD (temporomandibular joint dysfunction) has often been treated as a structural problem of the jaw and surrounding tissues. Treatment has included a mouthguard at night to prevent grinding of the teeth, braces, or surgical intervention to correct jaw malalignment. However, there is growing recognition that oftentimes there are no significant structural abnormalities of the jaw. Many clinicians now believe that TMD is a head-and-neck form of localized FM or myofascial pain. In 1992, diagnostic criteria for TMD suggested key symptoms to include recurrent facial or jaw pain and/or limitation in jaw opening occurring regularly over the past 6 months.[10] Ninety percent of FM patients report jaw and facial pain and many meet criteria for TMD (**Table 3.2**).

Irritable bladder and interstitial cystitis have also been reported with high frequency in FM.[13] The diagnosis of interstitial cystitis suggested by a 1987 conference recommended >9 months of bladder pain, urinary urgency and frequency, including voiding >8 times during the day and >2 times during the night, as well as a negative urine culture for infection.[8] Dysmenorrhea and unexplained chronic pelvic pain are also found commonly in patients with FM.

Not only is there a high occurrence of these variable functional illnesses with FM, their comorbidity has adverse consequences for the patient's overall health. Patients with both FM and CFS were more likely to be unemployed and see multiple health care providers compared with a patient diagnosed only with FM. They also have had worse overall health status and less satisfaction with their health care.

The comorbidity of FM with these other functional illnesses can be explained in a number of different ways. The pathophysiology of disorders, such as CFS, IBS, and musculoskeletal headaches, can be very similar to those of FM, as discussed in Chapter 5, *Pathophysiology*.[14] There is also significant overlap in case definitions for the functional somatic syndrome. For example, headache, fatigue, and abdominal pain are suggested clinical criteria for a number of these disorders. Furthermore, each of these disorders overlaps with both mood disturbances and multiple unexplained somatic symptoms. However, the majority of patients with these functional illnesses do not meet criteria for any single psychiatric diagnosis. The most logical explanation for the overlap of these functional illnesses is based on a better understanding of CNS dysregulation.

REFERENCES

1. Komaroff AL, Fagioli LR, Geiger AM, et al. An examination of the working case definition of chronic fatigue syndrome. *Am J Med.* 1996;100(1):56-64.

2. Aaron LA, Buchwald D. A review of the evidence for overlap among unexplained clinical conditions. *Ann Intern Med.* 2001;134(9 Pt 2):868-881.

3. Sharpe M. Chronic fatigue syndrome. *Psychiatr Clin North Am.* 1996;19(3):549-573.

4. Beard GM. Neurasthenia, or nervous exhaustion. *Boston Med Surg J.* 1869;3:217-221.

5. Fukuda K, Straus SE, Hickie I, Sharpe MC, Dobbins JG, Komaroff A. The chronic fatigue syndrome: a comprehensive approach to its definition and study. International Chronic Fatigue Syndrome Study Group. *Ann Intern Med.* 1994;121(12):953-959.

6. Goldenberg DL, Simms RW, Geiger A, Komaroff AL. High frequency of fibromyalgia in patients with chronic fatigue seen in a primary care practice. *Arthritis Rheum.* 1990;33(3):381-387.

7. Drossman DA. Diagnosing and treating patients with refractory functional gastrointestinal disorders. *Ann Intern Med.* 1995;123(9):688-697.

8. Kurland JE, Coyle WJ, Winkler A, Zable E. Prevalence of irritable bowel syndrome and depression in fibromyalgia. *Dig Dis Sci.* 2006;51(3):454-460.

9. Slotkoff AT, Radulovic DA, Clauw DJ. The relationship between fibromyalgia and the multiple chemical sensitivity syndrome. *Scand J Rheumatol.* 1997;26(5):364-367.

10. Aaron LA, Buchwald D. Chronic diffuse musculoskeletal pain, fibromyalgia and co-morbid unexplained clinical conditions. *Best Pract Res Clin Rheumatol.* 2003;17(4):563-574.

11. Goldenberg DL. Fibromyalgia, chronic fatigue syndrome, and myofascial pain. *Curr Opin Rheumatol.* 1996;8(2):113-123.

12. Wolfe F, Simon D, Fricton J, et al. The fibromyalgia and myofascial pain syndromes: a study of tender points and trigger points in persons with fibromyalgia, myofascial pain syndrome and no disease. *Arthritis Rheum.* 1990;33(9):S137.

13. Clauw DJ. Elusive syndromes: treating the biologic basis of fibromyalgia and related syndromes. *Cleve Clin J Med.* 2001;68(10):830, 832-834.

14. Clauw DJ, Chrousos GP. Chronic pain and fatigue syndromes: overlapping clinical and neuroendocrine features and potential pathogenic mechanisms. *Neuroimmunomodulation.* 1997;4(3):134-153.

4

Association With Mood, Cognitive, and Sleep Disturbances

It is not surprising that many clinicians have concluded that FM is a psychiatric illness or a manifestation of psychophysiologic abnormalities. Patients look well and there are no objective findings to account for the chronic symptoms based on the physical examination, laboratory results, or radiologic findings. Furthermore, many patients do report depression, anxiety, and high levels of stress. Indeed, each of the common functional illnesses discussed in Chapter 3, *Associated Illnesses*, overlap with mood disturbances, particularly with depression (**Figure 4.1**).

Pain comprises both physical and emotional responses. Higher rates of psychiatric disorders have been reported in all chronic pain conditions, including headaches and idiopathic low back pain. The nature of the cause-and-effect relationship between psychiatric disorders, especially depression, and chronic pain is unclear. It is possible that depression may be a consequence of any chronic pain disorder but we also know that depression frequently precedes the onset of pain symptoms. For example, one of the strongest predictors of developing FM prospectively has been self-reported depression at baseline.[1] Women who reported depressive symptoms were >6 times as likely to develop FM when compared with those who did not report depression. This suggests that depression and chronic pain may share a common pathway.

Multiple studies have demonstrated a higher rate of psychiatric disorders in FM patients compared with the general population. However, FM is not a psychiatric illness. At the time of the diagnosis of FM, mood disturbances are present in 30% to 50% of patients with FM (**Table 4.1**).[2] There are far greater odds of depressive illness (**Table 4.2**) and anxiety disorders (**Table 4.3**) in individuals with FM than in healthy controls.[3,4] There is

41

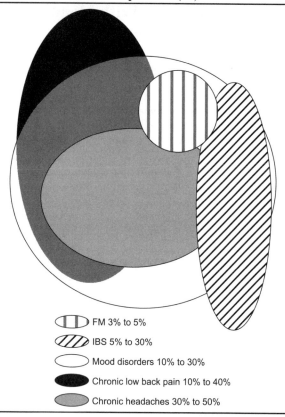

FM 3% to 5%

IBS 5% to 30%

Mood disorders 10% to 30%

Chronic low back pain 10% to 40%

Chronic headaches 30% to 50%

evidence to suspect shared biologic and genetic factors in
FM and depression, and there is coaggregation of FM and
mood disturbances (**Table 4.1**).[4] There is also a greater
personal and family history of mood disturbances in FM
compared with RA (**Table 4.4**).

The higher rate of psychiatric illness in FM is
especially prominent in patients who consult tertiary-
care physicians. For example, the current and lifetime
prevalence of depression or any mood disorder was
significantly greater for FM patients attending a specialty
clinic compared with the general population (**Figure
4.2**).[5] Investigators from the University of Alabama

TABLE 4.1 — Fibromyalgia and Mood Disorders

- At the time of FM diagnosis, mood disorders are present in 30% to 50%, primarily depression
- Increased prevalence of mood disorders is primarily in tertiary-referral patients
- Increased lifetime and family history of mood disorders in FM vs RA (OR 2.0)
- FM coaggregates with major mood disorder in families (OR 1.8 [95% CI 1.1, 2.9), $P=0.01$)

Arnold LM, et al. *J Clin Psychiatry*. 2006;67:1219-1225; Arnold LM, et al. *Arthritis Rheum*. 2004;50:944-952.

4

TABLE 4.2 — Co-occurrence of Fibromyalgia With Mood Disorders

	OR (95% CI) (Probands and Relatives Combined)	P Value
Major depression	2.7 (1.2-6.0)	0.013
Major mood disorder	6.2 (2.9-14)	<0.001

Arnold LM, et al. *J Clin Psychiatry*. 2006;67:1219-1225; Arnold LM, et al. *Arthritis Rheum*. 2004;50:944-952.

TABLE 4.3 — Co-occurrence of Fibromyalgia With Anxiety Disorders

	OR (95% CI) (Probands and Relatives Combined)	P Value
GAD	0.87 (0.21-3.7)	0.86
OCD	14 (2.8-72)	0.001
Panic disorder	5 (1.9-13)	0.001
PTSD	12 (2.9-51)	<0.001
Social phobia	8.9 (2.2-36)	0.002
Any anxiety disorder	6.7 (2.3-20)	<0.001

Arnold LM, et al. *J Clin Psychiatry*. 2006;67:1219-1225; Arnold LM, et al. *Arthritis Rheum*. 2004;50:944-952.

compared patients with FM with people in the community who had symptoms of FM but were not being followed for the condition (so-called nonpatients) and to healthy community controls.[6] The FM patients had a significantly

TABLE 4.4 — Lifetime Prevalence of Mood Disorders in Relatives of 78 Probands With Fibromyalgia and 40 Probands With Rheumatoid Arthritis

	Relatives of Probands	
	With FM (N=533) N (%)	With RA (N=272) N (%)
MDD	157 (29.5)	50 (18.3)
Bipolar I disorder	7 (1.3)	1 (0.4)
Bipolar II disorder	7 (1.3)	1 (0.4)
Any major mood disorder	171 (32.1)	52 (19.1)

Arnold LM, et al. *Arthritis Rheum*. 2004;50:944-952.

FIGURE 4.2 — Psychiatric Disorders in Patients With and Without Fibromyalgia and in Controls

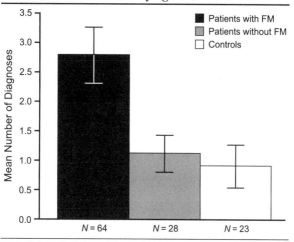

Aaron LA, et al. *Arthritis Rheum*. 1996;39:436-445.

greater number of lifetime psychiatric diagnoses than the nonpatients, who did not differ significantly from controls (**Figure 4.2**). The patients also had higher levels of psychological distress. Similar observations have been noted in patients with IBS.

The overlap of FM with somatization disorder is controversial. Somatization disorder is thought to be related to a maladaptive preoccupation with physical symptoms not associated with objective organ disease. It is likely that many patients with chronic illnesses of various types, including FM, have heightened somatic concerns and a maladaptive illness behavior, even if they do not meet the criteria for somatization disorder. In a prospective study of chronic widespread pain (CWP), 1953 adults aged between 18 and 69 were recruited from a population and completed a detailed pain questionnaire, which included a pain drawing as well as psychosocial instruments.[7] These studies were repeated 1 year later. After adjustment for age, sex, and pain category, there were strong relationships between baseline test scores and subsequent risk of CWP (**Table 4.5**). Those subjects free of CWP at baseline were at increased future risk for development of pain if they displayed aspects of somatization. The problem, however, is in the very nature of the concept of somatization, which could be viewed as simply a proxy for preexisting stress and mood disturbances.

TABLE 4.5 — Psychiatric Disorders in Patients With Regional and Widespread Pain

Disorder	No Pain (N=86) N (%)	Other Pain (N=143) N (%)	CWP (N=67) N (%)
Mood[a]	14 (16)	22 (15)	20 (30)
Anxiety[a]	12 (14)	25 (17)	14 (21)
Somatoform	0 (–)	1 (0.7)	2 (3)
Other	1 (1)	5 (3)	4 (6)
Total	23 (27)	41 (29)	30 (45)

[a] Includes subjects with diagnoses in >1 group of disorders.

McBeth J, et al. *Arthritis Rheum.* 2001;44:940-946.

As discussed in Chapter 5, *Pathophysiology*, stress may be a common pathway for chronic pain and mood disorders. There has also commonly been a history of increased physical and emotional trauma, including sexual abuse in childhood, in FM patients.[8] There have been numerous studies that have demonstrated an association between unexplained pelvic pain and IBS, as well as FM, with physical or sexual abuse in childhood. The range of childhood abuse in women with FM has been between 17% and 65%, although in some studies, this was not statistically higher than in the control population. These FM patients were also more likely to have a diagnosis of somatization disorder.

The presence of mood disorders also adversely affects the level of symptoms and the outcome of patients with FM. Self-assessed depression is a risk factor for the development of FM in women.[1] High levels of depression and anxiety are associated with more physical symptoms, greater overall ill health, and more dissatisfaction with health, interference from pain, and life stress.[9] The number of reported medical symptoms is positively associated with current and past depressive and anxiety disorders.[10] Patients with FM and concurrent depression are more likely to have difficulties in activities of daily living, perceive a greater degree of interference in their life associated with pain, and have less control because of the pain. However, no differences have been observed in pain severity or in the number of tender points between depressed and nondepressed FM patients.

Cognitive disturbances are prominent in FM as well as in depression, with a prevalence of 40% to 95% in FM patients (**Table 4.6**).[11] Katz and Leavitt found memory decline in 70% of FM patients vs 25% of other rheumatology patients and mental confusion in 40% vs 3.5%.[12] FM patients often describe "fibrofog"; common descriptions

TABLE 4.6 — Cognitive Problems in Fibromyalgia

- Cognitive difficulties in FM vs other rheumatology patients:[a]
  - Memory decline (70% vs 25%)
  - Mental confusion (40% vs 3.5%)
- Metamemory in FM patients:[b]
  - Lower memory capacity
  - More memory deterioration
  - Low self-efficacy over memory performance
  - Higher anxiety about memory
  - More strategy use

[a] Katz RS, et al. *J Clin Rheumatol*. 2004;10:53-58.
[b] Glass JM, et al. *J Psychosom Res*. 2005;58:263-269.

include "I have a significant decrease in my memory," "I used to be bright and quick but now am out of it," and, "I thought I had aphasia." Cognitive test abnormalities have been somewhat different in FM patients compared with those who have major depression.[11] In FM patients, common cognitive problems include task switching and rule-complexity testing (**Figure 4.3**).[13]

FIGURE 4.3 — Effects of Task Switching and Rule Complexity in Fibromyalgia vs Healthy Controls

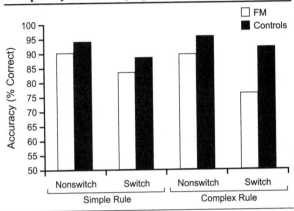

FM less accurate; $P=0.004$. Patient group by Switch by Rule Complexity Interaction $P=0.028$.

Glass JM, et al. *J Psychosom Res*. 2005;58(3):263-269.

FM patients and patients with mood disturbances also share abnormal sleep patterns. The most prominent sleep abnormality in FM patients is alpha-wave intrusion in stage IV sleep. Moldofsky and associates first demonstrated this in 1975 and produced FM-like symptoms in healthy subjects by arousing them from stage IV sleep (**Figure 4.4**).[14] Alpha intrusion during sleep can be of different patterns; phasic alpha activity (simultaneous with delta activity) correlated best with FM symptoms.[15] Periodic limb movements and sleep apnea may also complicate FM.[15] Circadian rhythms of women with FM do not differ from those of healthy controls.[16]

The close association of FM with mood disturbances mandates that every new FM patient be carefully

FIGURE 4.4 — Arousal Disturbances With Disruption of Slow-Wave (Deep) Sleep Caused Muscular Pain and Fatigue and Increased Sensitivity to Pain

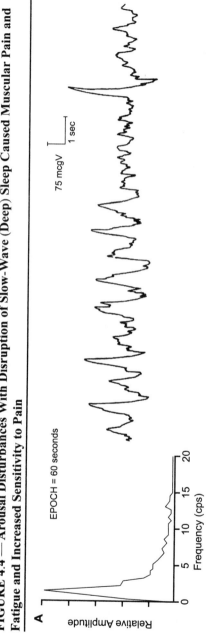

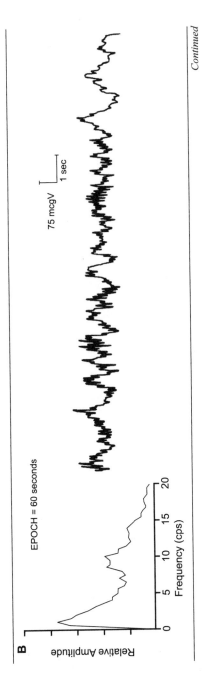

EPOCH = 60 seconds

75 mcgV

1 sec

Relative Amplitude

Frequency (cps)

0 5 10 15 20

B

Continued

49

FIGURE 4.4 — *Continued*

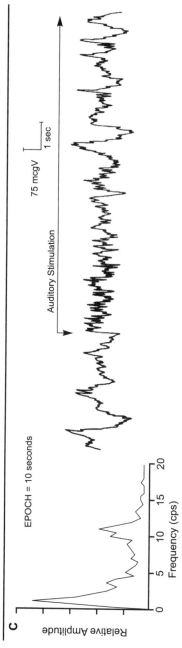

C
EPOCH = 10 seconds

Relative Amplitude

Frequency (cps)

Auditory Stimulation

75 mcgV
1 sec

Frequency spectra and raw EEG from *(A)* NREM (stage 4) sleep in a healthy 25-year-old subject. The spectrum shows that most amplitude is concentrated at 1 cps (delta). *(B)* NREM sleep in a 42-year-old "fibrositis" patient. The spectrum shows amplitude of both 1 cps (delta) and 8 to 10 cps (alpha). *(C)* NREM sleep of a healthy 21-year-old subject during stage 4 sleep deprivation. In the EEG, there is a clear association between external arousal (auditory stimulation) and alpha onset. Again the frequency spectrum (obtained by 10-second analysis from stimulus onset) shows amplitude concentrated in the delta and alpha bands.

Moldofsky H, et al. *Psychosom Med.* 1975;37:341-351.

evaluated for comorbidity of psychiatric illness. Even in patients with no psychiatric diagnosis, levels of psychosocial stressors, coping ability, and locus of control should be ascertained. Often this will require formal referral to a mental health professional.

In conclusion, FM and mood disorders coaggregate in families, suggesting common, heritable, and causal factors (**Table 4.7**). As discussed in *Chapter 5*, central monoaminergic neurotransmission is involved in mood regulation as well as in descending pain pathways. Dysfunction of the stress axis likely affects the development of mood disorders and FM. Chronic stress induces cytokine expression in the brain; cytokines, in turn, may contribute to symptoms of depression and pain enhancement.

TABLE 4.7 — Possible Etiologic Links Between Mood Disorders and Fibromyalgia

- FM and mood disorders coaggregate in families, suggesting common, possibly heritable, causal factors
- Central monoaminergic neurotransmission is involved in mood regulation and descending pain pathways
- Dysfunction of the HPA axis may contribute to the development of mood disorders and FM
- Chronic stress induces cytokine expression in the brain; cytokines, in turn, may contribute to symptoms of depression and pain enhancement

REFERENCES

1. Forseth KO, Førre O, Gran JT. A 5.5 year prospective study of self-reported musculoskeletal pain and of fibromyalgia in a female population: significance and natural history. *Clin Rheumatol.* 1999;18(2):114-121.

2. Goldenberg DL. Fibromyalgia syndrome a decade later: what have we learned? *Arch Intern Med.* 1999;159(8):777-785.

3. Arnold LM, Hudson JI, Hess EV, et al. Family study of fibromyalgia. *Arthritis Rheum.* 2004;50(3):944-952.

4. Arnold LM, Hudson JI, Keck PE, Auchenbach MB, Javaras KN, Hess EV. Comorbidity of fibromyalgia and psychiatric disorders. *J Clin Psychiatry.* 2006;67(8):1219-1225.

5. Epstein SA, Kay G, Clauw D, et al. Psychiatric disorders in patients with fibromyalgia. A multicenter investigation. *Psychosomatics.* 1999;40(1):57-63.

6. Aaron LA, Bradley LA, Alarcón GS, et al. Psychiatric diagnoses in patients with fibromyalgia are related to health care-seeking behavior rather than to illness. *Arthritis Rheum*. 1996;39(3):436-445.

7. McBeth J, Macfarlane GJ, Benjamin S, Silman AJ. Features of somatization predict the onset of chronic widespread pain: results of a large population-based study. *Arthritis Rheum*. 2001;44(4):940-946.

8. Hudson JI, Pope HG Jr. Does childhood sexual abuse cause fibromyalgia? *Arthritis Rheum*. 1995;38(2):161-163.

9. White KP, Nielson WR, Harth M, Ostbye T, Speechley M. Chronic widespread musculoskeletal pain with or without fibromyalgia: psychological distress in a representative community adult sample. *J Rheumatol*. 2002;29(3):588-594.

10. Walker EA, Keegan D, Gardner G, Sullivan M, Katon WJ, Bernstein D. Psychosocial factors in fibromyalgia compared with rheumatoid arthritis: I. Psychiatric diagnoses and functional disability. *Psychosom Med*. 1997;59(6):565-571.

11. Glass JM, Park DC. Cognitive dysfunction in fibromyalgia. *Curr Rheumatol Rep*. 2001;3(2):123-127.

12. Katz RS, Leavitt F. The effect of dissociation (an information processing deficit) on medical symptoms in rheumatic disease patients with and without fibromyalgia. *Arthritis Rheum*. 2002;46:S107.

13. Glass JM, Park DC, Minear M, Crofford LJ. Memory beliefs and function in fibromyalgia patients. *J Psychosom Res*. 2005;58(3): 263-269.

14. Moldofsky H, Scarisbrick P, England R, Smythe H. Musculo-sketal symptoms and non-REM sleep disturbance in patients with "fibrositis syndrome" and healthy subjects. *Psychosom Med*. 1975;37(4):341-351.

15. Burns JW, Crofford LJ, Chervin RD. Sleep stage dynamics in fibromyalgia patients and controls. *Sleep Med*. 2008;9(6):689-696.

16. Crofford LJ, Young EA, Engleberg NC, et al. Basal circadian and pulsatile ACTH and cortisol secretion in patients with fibromyalgia and/or chronic fatigue syndrome. *Brain Behav Immun*. 2004;18(4):314-325.

5 Pathophsiology

FM was initially thought to be an inflammatory pain disorder of the muscle. When that theory was discounted, FM was included in textbook chapters entitled soft-tissue rheumatism or nonarticular rheumatism. However, our current understanding of FM is focused on CNS pain dysregulation (**Table 5.1**).[1] There have been no clear signs of degeneration, regeneration, or inflammation in muscle tissue. No differences were noted in the levels of phosphocreatine, inorganic phosphate, and intracellular pH of the upper trapezius and tibialis anterior muscles after exercise in 13 women with FM and 13 sedentary control females, using phosphorus magnetic resonance spectroscopy (**Figure 5.1**).[2] Dynamic muscle strength and isometric muscle strength are similar to that in controls matched for the level of exercise. Most investigators now believe that any intrinsic muscle abnormalities in FM are secondary to inactivity and pain.[3]

Genetic studies, the associated disorders that cluster with FM, and new pathophysiologic investigations all suggest that FM is a disorder of augmented pain regulation (**Table 5.1**). As noted earlier, FM is closely linked with other pain disorders, such as IBS, vulvodynia, chronic headaches, and irritable bladder, and these do not necessarily involve skeletal muscle. Each of these conditions is also associated with widespread hyperalgesia. Furthermore, patients with FM have heightened sensitivity to numerous physical stressors, not just to pressure over muscle. For example, FM patients are sensitive to auditory stimuli, suggesting a global CNS augmentation in sensory processing.[4]

Genetic Predisposition

In a landmark family study on FM, Arnold and coworkers recruited FM patients and RA patients, along with at least one first-degree relative, from consecutive referrals to two community rheumatology outpatient prac-

**TABLE 5.1 — Fibromyalgia:
Pathophysiologic Pathways**

- Genetic factors:
  - 8 times more common in families
  - No single gene (COMT, 5-HTT haplotype)
- Triggers:
  - Infection
  - Physical
  - Emotional trauma
- Pathophysiologic mechanisms:
  - Central pain augmentation
  - Disordered sensory processing
  - Autonomic/neuroendocrine dysfunction

tices.[5] All patients and first-degree relatives were given the Structured Clinical Interview for *DSM-IV* (SCID) and a supplemental interview in SCID format regarding migraine, IBS, CFS, and FM, as well as the Family Interview for Genetic Studies (FIGS). Their pressure-pain threshold was measured with a dolorimeter. This study found that FM was strongly familial, with an odds ratio of 8.5 for first-degree relatives (**Table 5.2**). Furthermore, FM in probands was associated with decreased pressure pain threshold in their relatives. This study supports other observations that genetic factors are involved in etiology of FM as well as in general pain sensitivity. This study and others have also found a strong family aggregation of FM with mood disturbances and other chronic functional illnesses, such as IBS and CFS. Therefore, it makes sense to search for specific genetic factors in FM.

Unfortunately, at this time, there are no strong associations with a single candidate gene in large subsets of FM patients (**Table 5.2**). There have been reports of an association with the 5-HT_{2A} receptor polymorphism T/T phenotype as well as with haplotypes of the serotonin transporter gene.[6,7] A number of groups have looked specifically at the variability in the catechol-*O*-methyl-transferase (COMT) genotype in FM, since it has been linked to pain sensitivity in the general population.[8] Subjects with specific COMT haplotypes (eg, those that are experimentally associated with high pain sensitivity) are more likely to develop TMJD (**Figure 5.2**).[9] Pain

FIGURE 5.1 — No Evidence of Abnormal Muscle Metabolism in NMR Spectroscopy in Fibromyalgia vs Controls

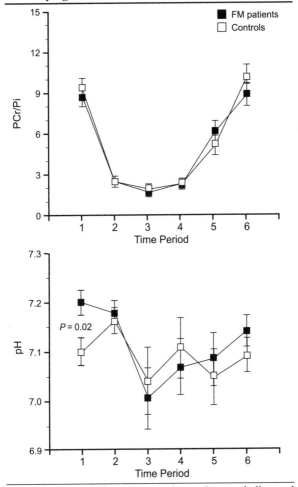

Demonstrates no difference in phosphocreatine metabolism and pH in FM vs controls.

Modified from: Simms RW, et al. *Arthritis Rheum.* 1994;37:794-800.

TABLE 5.2 — Genetics of Fibromyalgia

- A strong familial predisposition study by Arnold et al found[a]:
  - OR >8 for first-degree relatives
  - OR 2 for familial aggregation with:
    - Affective disorders
    - Bipolar
    - OCD
- Genes that may be involved in FM:
  - $5-HT_{2A}$ receptor polymorphism T/T phenotype[b]
  - Serotonin transporter[c]
  - Dopamine D4 receptor exon III repeat polymorphism[d]
  - COMT[e]

[a] Arnold LM, et al. *Arthritis Rheum.* 2004;50:944-952.
[b] Bondy B, et al. *Neurobiol Dis.* 1999;6:433-439.
[c] Offenbaecher M, et al. *Arthritis Rheum.* 1999;42:2482-2488.
[d] Buskila D, et al. *Mol Psychiatry.* 2004;9:730-731.
[e] Gürsoy S, et al. *Rheumatol Int.* 2003;23:104-107.

FIGURE 5.2 — Temporomandibular Joint Disorder Incidence Rates for COMT Haplotypes and Experimental Pain Groups

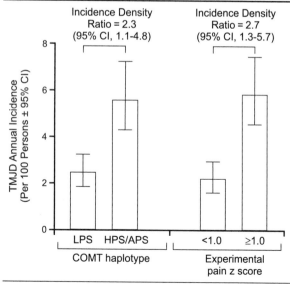

Based on: Diatchenko L, et al. *Hum Mol Genet.* 2005;14:135-143.

sensitivity in the general population follows a typical bell-shaped curve. There is a small percentage of the population who demonstrate heightened pain sensitivity which is likely related to both genetic and environmental factors.

As noted earlier, patients identify a number of stressors that trigger the onset of FM. These are often subclassified into physical, emotional, and infectious factors. Motor vehicle accidents, especially those involving the head and neck, have been capable of precipitating FM in a number of studies.[10] Infections, including nonspecific viral infections or Lyme disease, and varieties of psychological distress have also precipitated the disorder. Certain medications, such as the withdrawal of steroids, anecdotally have been associated with the onset of FM.

Central Pain Augmentation

The current thinking regarding the pathophysiology of FM integrates pain augmentation in the CNS with altered neuroendocrine and autonomic nervous system function. There is significant evidence for heightened sensitivity of peripheral and CNS pain pathways in FM. FM is manifest by both regional and widespread hyperalgesia and allodynia. FM patients demonstrate normal detection to sensory stimuli but uniformly have decreased threshold to noxious stimuli, which includes pressure, electrical, and heat sensations, as well as auditory stimuli. This reaction is independent of psychological factors.

An elegant series of experiments have demonstrated abnormal temporal summation of pain, referred to as "wind up," in FM.[11] Patients with FM demonstrate an exaggerated secondary response in muscle to painful stimuli from persistent peripheral C-fiber firing. This can be linked to specific areas of the brain involved with pain processing (**Figure 5.3**). This secondary pain response in the dorsal horn activates the N-methyl-D-aspartate (NMDA) receptor. The NMDA receptor antagonist ketamine has been utilized successfully for pain reduction in FM.[7]

There is good evidence for abnormalities in the descending analgesic pathway in FM (**Table 5.3**). The

FIGURE 5.3 — Pain Augmentation: Wind Up

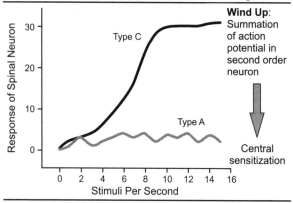

TABLE 5.3 — Alterations in Descending Analgesic Activity in Fibromyalgia

Opioids
- Normal or high levels of CSF enkephalins[a]
- Never administered in RCT, but most feel that opioids are ineffective or marginally effective
- Harris recently used PET to show decreased mu-opioid receptor binding in FM[b]

Noradrenergic/Serotoninergic
- Elevated levels of substance P in CSF in FM[c]
- Nearly any class of drug that raises *both* serotonin and norepinephrine levels has demonstrated efficacy in FM

[a] Baraniuk JN, et al. *BMC Musculoskelet Disord.* 2004;5:48.
[b] Harris JA, et al. *J Neurosci.* 2007;27:7136-7140.
[c] Russell IJ, et al. *Arthritis Rheum.* 1992;35:550-556.

level of substance P in the CSF was 3-fold higher in FM patients than in normal controls.[12] The regional cerebral blood flow, as detected by single photon emission computed tomography, was reduced in the left and right hemithalami, the right heads of the caudate nuclei, and pontine tegmentum in FM compared with controls.[13] There are normal or high levels of cerebrospinal fluid (CSF) enkephalins in FM.[14] This may explain the relative ineffectiveness of opioids in FM. Positron emission tomography (PET) scans demonstrated decreased mu-opioid receptor binding in FM.[15]

The most robust evidence for CNS pain dysregulation in FM is from recent brain imaging, using functional magnetic resonance imaging (fMRI) or PET scanning. These studies clearly demonstrate increased activity in both the sensory and the affective areas of the brain in FM patients compared with control subjects (**Figure 5.4, Table 5.4**). This has included evidence of hypoperfusion of the thalamus and head of the caudate nucleus and fMRI evidence of augmentated pain perception with increased activity in the somatosensory cortex and the insula.[16-18] In FM, levels of depression did not modulate the sensory aspects of pain but correlated with the magnitude of brain activation in the medial region of the brain. Catastrophizing correlated with pain response in these medial brain regions.

Dynamic changes in posterior insula glutamate concentration were also found in PET scans (**Figure 5.5**).[19] Brain gray matter, white matter, CSF, and total volume were compared in 10 FM patients and 10 healthy control subjects (**Figure 5.6**).[20] The FM patients demonstrated significant gray matter loss, with 1 year of FM pain equivalent to 9 years of brain aging.

The Neuroendocrine System and Stress

There is evidence for neuroendocrine dysfunction in FM.[1,21] This fits with theories of stress susceptibility as determined by genetic, environmental, and physiologic factors. Such a model correlates with the increased incidence of physical and psychological abuse in individuals who develop FM and related conditions, such as CFS and IBS. It also fits with FM following posttraumatic stress disorder (PTSD) or after a motor vehicle accident.

The hypothalamic-pituitary-adrenal (HPA) axis links pain and other stressors to endocrine, autonomic, and behavioral responses (**Figure 5.7**). Specific neuroendocrine findings have included low 24-hour urinary free cortisol, an exaggerated adrenocorticotropic hormone (ACTH) response to corticotropic-releasing hormone (CRH), a decreased net CRH response to CRH, and altered epinephrine and norepinephrine response to stressors,[22] (**Figure 5.7**). There is some evidence for a

FIGURE 5.4 — Brain Regional Blood Flow Response to Pain in Fibromyalgia vs Controls

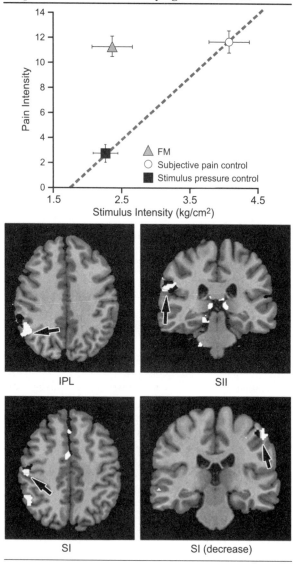

IPL

SII

SI

SI (decrease)

Continued

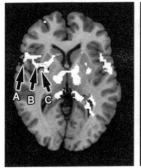
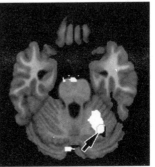

(A) STG, *(B)* Insula,
(C) Putamen

Cerebellum

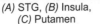

Gracely RH, et al. *Arthritis Rheum.* 2002;46:1333-1343.

TABLE 5.4 — Neuroimaging in Fibromyalgia

- Hypoperfusion of thalamus and head of the caudate nucleus
- fMRI of cortical response to pain consistent with augmentated pain perception
- In FMS, levels of depression did not modulate the sensory aspects of pain but correlated with the magnitude of brain activation in the medial region of the brain
- Catastrophizing correlated with pain response in these medial brain regions
- Changes in posterior insular glutamate in PET scans

Gracely RH, et al. *Arthritis Rheum.* 2002;46:1333-1343; Giesecke T, et al. *Arthritis Rheum.* 2005;52:1577-1584; Harris RE, et al. *Arthritis Rheum.* 2008;58:903-907.

---

functional reduction in serotoninergic activity in patients with FM and lower serum serotonin concentration than healthy controls.[23] Crofford and coworkers found that the pattern of basal circadian and pulsatile ACTH and cortisol secretion in FM patients was different than in controls, consistent with loss of HPA axis resiliency.[21]

McBeth and colleagues have demonstrated that psychosocial factors and stress reactivity are important factors in determining who will develop CWP.[24] They prospectively evaluated 11,000 subjects and found that 768 were at risk for CWP because of their psychosocial

FIGURE 5.5 — Higher Glutamate Levels Associated With Increased Fibromyalgia Pain

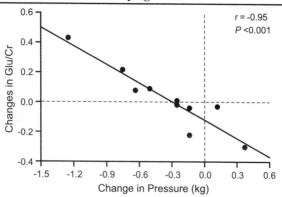

Patients with high insular glutamate had increased pain.

Adapted from: Harris RE, et al. *Arthritis Rheum*. 2008;58:903-907.

FIGURE 5.6 — Accelerated Brain Gray Matter Loss in Fibromyalgia

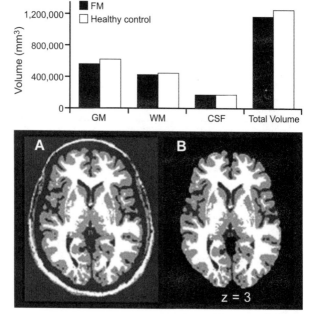

Continued

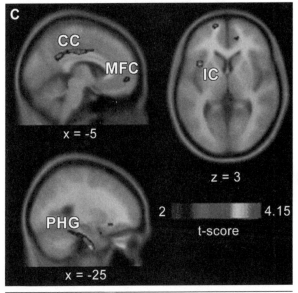

Brain gray matter, white matter, CSF, and total volume in 10 FM patients and 10 healthy control subjects.

Kuchinad A, et al. *J Neurosci*. 2007;27:4004-4007.

profile. There was a strong relationship of the HPA axis at baseline with developing CWP (**Figure 5.8**). The greater number of abnormal HPA studies at baseline directly increased the odds ratio of the patient developing persistent widespread pain.

Cytokines increase HPA and monoamine activity. Uceyler and colleagues found lower relative gene expression for interleukin (IL)-2 and lower levels of IL-4 and IL-10 in patients with CWP than in controls.[25] The lack of anti-inflammatory and analgesic Th2 cytokine activity was postulated to contribute to the pathogenesis of the CWP.

Increased skin hyperreactivity, cold sensitivity, and orthostatic intolerance noted in FM patients suggest alterations in the autonomic nervous system. Autonomic dysfunction has been demonstrated in a number of experimental studies, utilizing power spectral analysis to detect increased heart rate variability in women with FM compared with healthy, age-matched controls.[26,27]

FIGURE 5.7 — Neuroendocrine Studies in Fibromyalgia

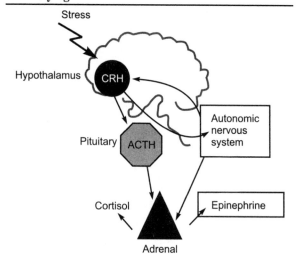

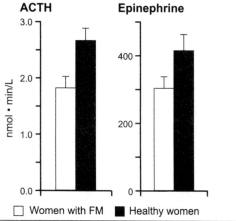

Low 24-hour urinary free cortisol; exaggerated ACTH response to CRH; decreased net CRH response to CRH; altered epinephrine, norepinephrine response to stressors. HPA axis links pain and other stressors to endocrine, autonomic, and behavioral responses.

Adler GK, et al. *Am J Med.* 1999;106:534-543.

FIGURE 5.8 — Odds of Developing Chronic Widespread Pain Based on Hypothalamic-Pituitary-Adrenal Function

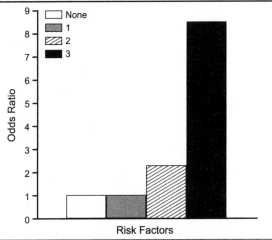

Based on none, 1, 2, or 3 risk factors: dexamethasone suppression test, morning cortisol, evening cortisol.

McBeth J, et al. *Arthritis Rheum.* 2007;56:360-371.

Others with FM have demonstrated orthostatic intolerance characterized by sympathetic hyperactivity and concomitantly reduced parasympathetic activity.[28,29]

There are abundant connections of the neuroendocrine and analgesic pathways (**Figure 5.9**). Neurotransmitters, including norepinephrine and 5-HT, mediate endogenous pain-inhibitory descending pathways. Dysfunction of these pathways is important in the lowered pain thresholds in FM patients.

REFERENCES

1. Clauw DJ, Crofford LJ. Chronic widespread pain and fibromyalgia: what we know, and what we need to know. *Best Pract Res Clin Rheumatol.* 2003;17(4):685-701.

2. Simms RW, Roy SH, Hrovat M, et al. Lack of association between fibromyalgia syndrome and abnormalities in muscle energy metabolism. *Arthritis Rheum.* 1994;37(6):794-800.

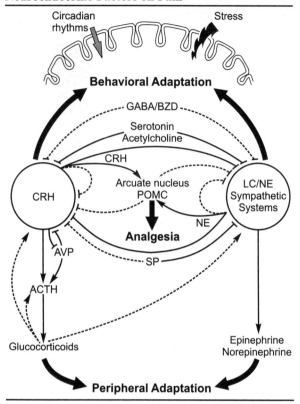

3. Simms RW. Fibromyalgia is not a muscle disorder. *Am J Med Sci.* 1998;315(6):346-350.

4. Geisser ME, Strader Donnell C, Petzke F, Gracely RH, Clauw DJ, Williams DA. Comorbid somatic symptoms and functional status in patients with fibromyalgia and chronic fatigue syndrome: sensory amplification as a common mechanism. *Psychosomatics.* 2008;49(3):235-242.

5. Arnold LM, Hudson JI, Hess EV, et al. Family study of fibromyalgia. *Arthritis Rheum.* 2004;50(3):944-952.

6. Bondy B, Spaeth M, Offenbaecher M, et al. The T102C polymorphism of the 5-HT2A-receptor gene in fibromyalgia. *Neurobiol Dis.* 1999;6(5):433-439.

7. Gürsoy S, Erdal E, Herken H, Madenci E, Alaşehirli B. Association of T102C polymorphism of the 5-HT2A receptor gene with psychiatric status in fibromyalgia syndrome. *Rheumatol Int.* 2001;21(2):58-61.

8. Buskila D, Sarzi-Puttini P. Biology and therapy of fibromyalgia. Genetic aspects of fibromyalgia syndrome. *Arthritis Res Ther.* 2006;8(5):218.

9. Diatchenko L, Slade GD, Nackley AG, et al. Genetic basis for individual variations in pain perception and the development of a chronic pain condition. *Hum Mol Genet.* 2005;14(1):135-143.

10. Buskila D, Neumann L, Vaisberg G, Alkalay D, Wolfe F. Increased rates of fibromyalgia following cervical spine injury. A controlled study of 161 cases of traumatic injury. *Arthritis Rheum.* 1997;40(3):446-452.

11. Staud R. Biology and therapy of fibromyalgia: pain in fibromyalgia syndrome. *Arthritis Res Ther.* 2006;8(3):208.

12. Russell IJ, Orr MD, Littman B, et al. Elevated cerebrospinal fluid levels of substance P in patients with the fibromyalgia syndrome. *Arthritis Rheum.* 1994;37(11):1593-1601.

13. Mountz JM, Bradley LA, Modell JG, et al. Fibromyalgia in women. Abnormalities of regional cerebral blood flow in the thalamus and the caudate nucleus are associated with low pain threshold levels. *Arthritis Rheum.* 1995;38(7):926-938.

14. Baraniuk JN, Whalen G, Cunningham J, Clauw DJ. Cerebrospinal fluid levels of opioid peptides in fibromyalgia and chronic low back pain. *BMC Musculoskelet Disord.* 2004;5:48.

15. Harris RE, Clauw DJ, Scott DJ, McLean SA, Gracely RH, Zubieta JK. Decreased central mu-opioid receptor availability in fibromyalgia. *J Neurosci.* 2007;27(37):10000-10006.

16. Gracely RH, Petzke F, Wolf JM, Clauw DJ. Functional magnetic resonance imaging evidence of augmented pain processing in fibromyalgia. *Arthritis Rheum.* 2002;46(5):1333-1343.

17. Gracely RH, Geisser ME, Giesecke T, et al. Pain catastrophizing and neural responses to pain among persons with fibromyalgia. *Brain.* 2004;127(Pt 4):835-843.

18. Giesecke T, Williams DA, Harris RE, et al. Subgrouping of fibromyalgia patients on the basis of pressure-pain thresholds and psychological factors. *Arthritis Rheum.* 2003;48(10):2916-2922.

19. Harris RE, Sundgren PC, Pang Y, et al. Dynamic levels of glutamate within the insula are associated with improvements in multiple pain domains in fibromyalgia. *Arthritis Rheum.* 2008;58(3):903-907.

20. Kuchinad A, Schweinhardt P, Seminowicz DA, Wood PB, Chizh BA, Bushnell MC. Accelerated brain gray matter loss in fibromyalgia patients: premature aging of the brain? *J Neurosci.* 2007;27(15):4004-4007.

21. Crofford LJ, Young EA, Engleberg NC, et al. Basal circadian and pulsatile ACTH and cortisol secretion in patients with fibromyalgia and/or chronic fatigue syndrome. *Brain Behav Immun.* 2004;18(4):314-325.

22. Adler GK, Kinsley BT, Hurwitz S, Mossey CJ, Goldenberg DL. Reduced hypothalamic-pituitary and sympathoadrenal responses to hypoglycemia in women with fibromyalgia syndrome. *Am J Med.* 1999;106(5):534-543.

23. Russell IJ. Neurochemical pathogenesis of fibromyalgia. *Z Rheumatol.* 1998;57(suppl 2):63-66.

24. McBeth J, Chiu YH, Silman AJ, et al. Hypothalamic-pituitary-adrenal stress axis function and the relationship with chronic widespread pain and its antecedents. *Arthritis Res Ther.* 2005;7(5):R992-R1000.

25. Uçeyler N, Valenza R, Stock M, Schedel R, Sprotte G, Sommer C. Reduced levels of antiinflammatory cytokines in patients with chronic widespread pain. *Arthritis Rheum.* 2006;54(8):2656-2664.

26. Martínez-Lavín M, Hermosillo AG, Rosas M, Soto ME. Circadian studies of autonomic nervous balance in patients with fibromyalgia: a heart rate variability analysis. *Arthritis Rheum.* 1998;41(11):1966-1971.

27. Martínez-Lavín M, Hermosillo AG. Autonomic nervous system dysfunction may explain the multisystem features of fibromyalgia. *Semin Arthritis Rheum.* 2000;29(4):197-199.

28. Ulas UH, Unlu E, Hamamcioglu K, Odabasi Z, Cakci A, Vural O. Dysautonomia in fibromyalgia syndrome: sympathetic skin responses and RR interval analysis. *Rheumatol Int.* 2006;26(5):383-387.

29. Bou-Holaigah I, Calkins H, Flynn JA, et al. Provocation of hypotension and pain during upright tilt table testing in adults with fibromyalgia. *Clin Exp Rheumatol.* 1997;15(3):239-246.

6 Pharmacologic Management

There are many reasons why medications that act primarily on the CNS have been the most effective in the treatment of FM (**Table 6.1**). As research studies found no evidence for significant pathologic abnormalities in the painful muscles of patients with FM, attention naturally shifted to pain augmentation mechanisms. Chapter 5, *Pathophysiology*, details the ever-expanding experimental evidence for altered neural pain processing in FM. Furthermore, the strong association with mood disturbances, sleep disturbances, cognitive disturbances, and exhaustion suggest a primary CNS disorder. Therefore, during the past 25 years, there has been a succession of analgesics, antidepressants, and antiseizure drugs utilized in clinical trials for the treatment of FM (**Table 6.2**).[1]

Until 2008, no drugs had been approved by the Food and Drug Administration (FDA) for the treatment of FM. However, in 2008, two medications, pregabalin and duloxetine, have been approved by the FDA.

Antiseizure Drugs: Pregabalin and Gabapentin

■ Pregabalin

The first drug approved by the FDA for the management of FM was pregabalin. Pregabalin was initially approved for the treatment of seizure disorders. It has been approved in the United States and Europe for adjunctive therapy for adult patients with partial onset seizures and for neuropathic pain. In the United States, pregabalin is approved for the management of neuropathic pain associated with diabetic peripheral neuropathy and postherpetic neuralgia; in Europe, for central neuropathic pain and generalized anxiety disorder.

Pregabalin and gabapentin both bind to the $\alpha2\delta$ subunit of voltage-gated calcium channels of neurons. Their analgesic action is possibly related to reduction of calcium influx at nerve terminals, inhibiting release

TABLE 6.1 — Rationale for the Use of Central Nervous System Active Medications in Fibromyalgia

- No evidence of muscle pathology
- Current research supports role of augmented central pain mechanisms:
  - Genetic predisposition:
    - $5-HT_{2A}$ receptor polymorphism
    - ↑ Pain severity in FM patients with T/T genotypes
    - ↑ Frequency of S/S genotype in FM patients compared with healthy controls
    - ↑ Incidence of COMT polymorphism in FM patients
  - Substance P increased in CSF
  - 5-HT and NE serum levels decreased in some studies
  - Imaging studies
- Elevated lifetime rates of mood disorders in patients with FM
- Elevated rates of mood disorders in first-degree relatives of FM patients
- Sleep disturbances

Russell IJ, et al. *Arthritis Rheum*. 1992;35:550-556; Bondy B, et al. *Neurobiol Dis*. 1999;6:433-439; Offenbaecher M, et al. *Arthritis Rheum*. 1999;42:2482-2488; Arnold LM, et al. *Arthritis Rheum*. 2004;50:944-952; Moldofsky H. *Adv Neuroimmunol*. 1995;5:39-56; Buskila D, Sarzi-Puttini P. *Arthritis Res Ther*. 2006;8:218; Harris RE, et al. *Arthritis Rheum*. 2008;58:903-907.

of neurotransmitters such as glutamate and substance P (**Figure 6.1**).[2] In the initial, randomized clinical trial (RCT), 529 FM patients were randomly assigned to 300, 450, and 600 mg of pregabalin or placebo (**Figure 6.2**).[2] Patients had to meet the ACR criteria for FM and score ≥4 on a daily pain diary (0–10) at baseline and score ≥40 on the Visual Analog Scale (VAS; 0–100 mm) of the Short-Form McGill Pain Questionnaire (SF-MPQ) at screening and randomization. The characteristics of these four patient groups were similar at baseline (**Table 6.3**). There was significant improvement in pain, at 450 mg/day, as well as global well-being, over 3 months compared with placebo (**Figure 6.3** and **Figure 6.4**). There was also improvement in sleep quality, fatigue, and health-related quality of life.

The two studies used to establish FDA approval of pregabalin in FM included a 14-week, double-blind, placebo-controlled, multicenter study[3] and one 6-month,

**TABLE 6.2 — Medicines Used in
Fibromyalgia Trials**

Drug Class	Agents	RCT Testing?
Antidepressants	SSRIs	+
	SNRIs	+
	TCAs	+
Analgesics	NSAIDs	+
	Tramadol	+
Muscle relaxants	Cyclobenzaprine	+
	Tizanidine	−
	Carisoprodol	−
	Methocarbamol	−
Sedative/hypnotics	Trazodone	−
	Zolpidem	+
	Zopiclone	+
	Sodium oxybate	+
	Pramipexole	+
Antiepileptics	Gabapentin	+
	Pregabalin	+

randomized withdrawal study.[4] Both studies enrolled patients with a diagnosis of FM using the ACR criteria (history of widespread pain for 3 months, and pain present at ≥11 of the 18 specific tender-point sites). Each of these studies showed a significant reduction in pain compared with placebo by the VAS. In addition, improvement was demonstrated based on PGIC and FIQ.

The initial 14-week study compared pregabalin at total daily doses of 300 mg, 450 mg, and 600 mg with placebo.[3] Patients were enrolled with a minimum mean baseline pain score of ≥4 on an 11-point numeric pain rating scale and a score of ≥40 mm on the 10-mm pain VAS. The baseline mean pain score in this trial was 6.7. Responders to placebo in an initial 1-week run-in phase were not randomized into subsequent phases of the study. A total of 64% of patients randomized to pregabalin completed the study.

There was statistically significant improvement in pain at 450 mg and 600 mg compared with placebo (**Figure 6.5** and **Figure 6.6**). There was no evidence of a greater effect on pain scores of the 600-mg daily dose than the 450-mg daily dose, but there was evidence of

FIGURE 6.1 — Pregabalin and Gabapentin

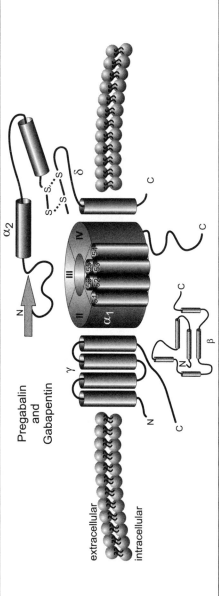

These drugs bind to α_2-δ subunit of voltage-gated calcium (C) channels of neurons (N), reducing calcium influx at nerve terminals and therefore inhibiting release of neurotransmitters, including glutamate and substance P.

Based on: Crofford LJ, et al. *Arthritis Rheum*. 2005;52:1264-1273.

FIGURE 6.2 — Initial Pregabalin in Fibromyalgia Study Design

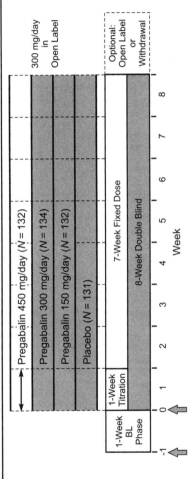

A randomized, double-blind, placebo-controlled trial (N = 529). Patients randomly assigned to receive 450 mg/day first received 300 mg/day for 3 days, receiving a fixed dose of 450 mg/day thereafter.

Crofford LJ, et al. *Arthritis Rheum.* 2005;52:1264-1273.

TABLE 6.3 — Demographic and Baseline Characteristics in First Pregabalin Trial

Characteristic	Placebo	Pregabalin		
		150 mg/day	300 mg/day	450 mg/day
Number of patients	131	132	134	132
Female (%)	90.8	95.5	89.6	90.2
Mean age (years)	49.7	48.0	47.7	48.9
Mean duration of FM (years)	≈8.6	≈8.5	≈9.2	≈9.6
Mean number of tender points at BL	17.2	17.0	17.3	16.8
BL mean pain score	6.9	6.9	7.3	7.0

FIGURE 6.3 — Pregabalin in Fibromyalgia: Mean Pain Scores

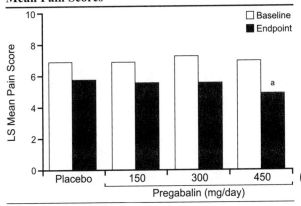

Crofford LJ, et al. *Arthritis Rheum.* 2005;52:1264-1273.

FIGURE 6.4 — Pregabalin in Fibromyalgia: Patient Global Impression of Change

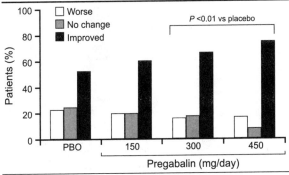

Crofford LJ, et al. *Arthritis Rheum.* 2005;52:1264-1273.

dose-dependent adverse reactions. Some patients experienced a decrease in pain as early as Week 1, which persisted throughout the study. The figure is cumulative. Patients who did not complete the study were assigned 0% improvement. Some patients experienced a decrease in pain as early as Week 1, which persisted throughout the study.

FIGURE 6.5 — Pain Improvement With Pregabalin in Fibromyalgia

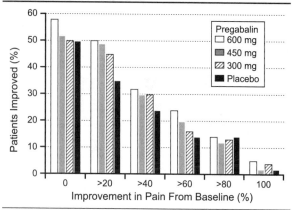

Arnold LM, et al. *J Pain.* 2008;9:792-805.

FIGURE 6.6 — Pain Improvement With Various Doses of Pregabalin in Fibromyalgia

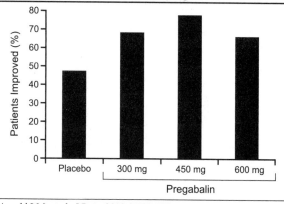

Arnold LM, et al. *J Pain.* 2008;9:792-805.

The second randomized withdrawal study compared pregabalin with placebo.[4] Patients were titrated during a 6-week open-label dose optimization phase to a total daily dose of 300 mg, 450 mg, or 600 mg. Patients were considered to be responders if they had both at least a 50% reduction in pain (VAS) and rated their overall improvement on the PGIC as much improved or very much improved. Those who responded to treatment were then randomized in the double-blind treatment phase to either the dose achieved in the open-label phase or to placebo. Patients were treated for up to 6 months following randomization. Efficacy was assessed by time to loss of therapeutic response, defined as either a <30% reduction in pain (VAS) from open-label baseline during two consecutive visits of the double-blind phase or a worsening of FM symptoms necessitating an alternative treatment. Fifty-four percent of patients were able to titrate to an effective and tolerable dose of pregabalin during the 6-week open-label phase. Of the patients entering the randomized treatment phase assigned to remain on pregabalin, 38% of patients completed 26 weeks of treatment vs 19% of placebo-treated patients (**Figure 6**.7).

6

FIGURE 6.7 — Time to Loss of Therapeutic Response to Pregabalin vs Placebo

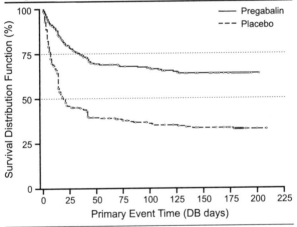

- Comparison of pregabalin with placebo in time to LTR (Kaplan-Meier log-rank test): P <0.0001
- LTR by end of DB:
  - Placebo: N=174 (61%)
  - Pregabalin: N=90 (32%)
  - Each of six sensitivity analyses confirmed the robustness of the primary analysis (all P <0.0001).

Crofford LJ, et al. *Pain*. 2008;136(3):419-431.

When considering return of pain or withdrawal due to adverse events as loss of response, treatment with pregabalin resulted in a longer time to loss of therapeutic response than treatment with placebo. Fifty-three percent of the pregabalin-treated subjects compared with 33% of placebo patients remained on study drug and maintained a therapeutic response to Week 26 of the study. Treatment with pregabalin also resulted in a longer time to loss of response based on the FIQ and longer time to loss of overall assessment of patient status as measured by the PGIC.

The most common adverse side effects in these two trials included somnolence, dizziness, fluid retention, and weight gain (**Figure 6.8**).[3,4] These side effects can be minimized by starting pregabalin at low doses and taking it in the evening.

The recommended dose of pregabalin for FM is 300 mg to 450 mg/day. The recommended starting dose according to the package insert is 75 mg twice daily, but some patients may have better compliance if lower doses, such as 50 mg at bedtime, are begun initially. Patients who do not experience sufficient benefit with 300 mg/day may be further increased to 225 mg two times a day (450 mg/day). Although pregabalin was also studied at 600 mg/day, there is no evidence that this dose confers additional benefit and this dose was less well tolerated. In view of the dose-dependent adverse reactions, treatment with doses >450 mg/day is not recommended. Because pregabalin is eliminated primarily by renal excretion, the dose should be adjusted for patients with reduced renal function.

■ **Gabapentin**

A single 12-week, double-blind, randomized study compared gabapentin in doses of 1200 to 2400 mg/day ($N = 75$) with placebo ($N = 75$).[5] The primary outcome measure was at least a 30% reduction in the Brief Pain Inventory (BPI) 24-hour average pain-severity score. The gabapentin-treated patients demonstrated significantly greater reduction in pain severity and interference from pain compared with the placebo-treated patients (**Figure 6.9**).

Furthermore, the gabapentin-treated patients had significantly greater global improvement and improvement in sleep and vitality, as well as reduction in the total impact of FM. The median dose was 1800 mg/day and the mean dose was 1682 mg/day. The adverse side effects were similar to those in the clinical trials with pregabalin.

Gabapentin is not approved by the FDA for the treatment of FM.

Serotonin-Norepinephrine Reuptake Inhibitors: Duloxetine and Milnacipran

■ Duloxetine

Duloxetine is the second drug approved by the FDA for the management of FM. The recommended dose is 60 mg once daily. Duloxetine is a dual serotonin-norepinephrine reuptake inhibitor (SNRI). Three antidepressants with dual serotonin and norepinephrine reuptake inhibition (venlafaxine, duloxetine, and milnacipran) have been evaluated in RCTs in FM. There have been one RCT and two open-label studies with venlafaxine (**Table 6.4**). There was no significant improvement in the single RCT, although the dose used may have been too small for any analgesic effect.[6]

Duloxetine has been evaluated in a number of clinical trials (**Table 6.5**). In two pivotal, 12-week studies involving 874 patients with FM, duloxetine was more effective than placebo in relieving pain based on changes in the BPI and 24-hour average pain scale (**Figure 6.10** and **Figure 6.11**).[7,8] Significant improvement in pain was noted in the first week of study and there was also improvement in global well-being and function. Significant improvement in pain for duloxetine vs placebo was observed in the first week of each study. Fifty-one percent and 55% of patients on duloxetine had a 30% improvement on the BPI at end point (at least 30% pain reduction is considered clinically meaningful). Duloxetine was also superior to placebo on the Fibromyalgia Impact Questionnaire (FIQ) total score, a scale that is used to assess and evaluate the impact of FM on aspects of health and functioning. In addition, 65% and 66% of patients taking duloxetine 60 mg daily reported feeling better at end point as measured by the Patient Global Impression of Improvement (PGI-I). The PGI-I is a patient-rated scale that evaluates how much

FIGURE 6.8 — Adverse Events in Pooled Trials With Pregabalin

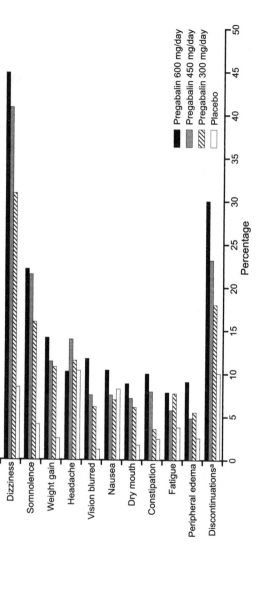

80

Among all pregabalin patients, dizziness (6.4%) and somnolence (4.0%) were the adverse events that most commonly led to discontinuation. Incidence of treatment-emergent adverse events tended to increase with dosage.

[a] Due to all-cause adverse events.

Arnold LM, et al. *Ann Rheum Dis*. 2007;66(suppl 2):62; Mease PJ, et al. *J Rheumatol*. 2008;35(3):502-514.

6

FIGURE 6.9 — 30% Reduction on Average Pain Severity Score With Gabapentin

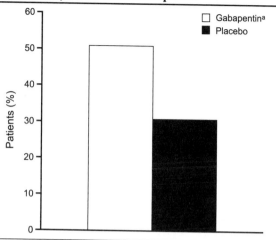

[a] $P = 0.014$.

Adapted from: Arnold LM, et al. *Arthritis Rheum.* 2007;56:1336-1344.

improvement has occurred since beginning treatment. The efficacy of duloxetine was independent of mood status (**Figure 6.12**). In four pooled studies, the most commonly observed adverse events in duloxetine-treated patients with FM (≥5% and at least twice that of placebo) were nausea (29%), dry mouth (18%), constipation (15%), decreased appetite (11%), sleepiness (11%), increased sweating (7%), and agitation (6%). In the placebo-controlled clinical trials, the overall discontinuation rates due to adverse events for duloxetine vs placebo were 20% and 12%, respectively (**Figure 6.13**).

In a 6-month, double-blind trial, duloxetine 60 mg/day and 120 mg/day were both superior to placebo on the BPI average pain score and the global change score at 3 months.[9] At 6 months, only duloxetine 120 mg/day was superior on both outcome measures (**Figure 6.14**).[8] Duloxetine is also approved for the treatment of major depressive disorder, diabetic peripheral neuropathic pain, and generalized anxiety disorder.

TABLE 6.4 — Venlafaxine: Clinical Trials in Fibromyalgia

Study	N	Dose (mg/day)	Treatment Duration (weeks)
Phase 2[a] *RCT*	90	75	6
Phase 2[b] *Open label*	15	37.5-300	8
Phase 2[c] *Open label*	15	75	12

[a] Zijsltra TR, et al. *Arthritis Rheum*. 2002;46:S105. Results in the RCT: no statistically significant improvements were found across pain, fatigue, sleep, depression, or general health.
[b] Dwight MM, et al. *Psychosomatics*. 1998;39:14-17.
[c] Sayar K, et al. *Ann Pharmacother*. 2003;37:1561-1565.

6

TABLE 6.5 — Duloxetine: Clinical Trials in Fibromyalgia

Study	N	Dose (mg/day)	Treatment Duration (weeks)
Phase 2[a] *+/– MDD*	207	120	12
Phase 3[b] *Females only +/– MDD*	354	60 120	12
Phase 3[c] *+/– MDD*	520	20 60 120	28
Phase 3[d] *+/– MDD*	330	60/120	27

[a] Arnold LM, et al. *Arthritis Rheum*. 2004;50:2974-2984.
[b] Arnold LM, et al. *Pain*. 2005;119:5-15.
[c] Russell IJ, et al. *Musculoskel Pain*. 2007;15(suppl 13):58.
[d] Russell IJ, et al. *Pain*. 2008;136:432-444.

■ Milnacipran

Milnacipran, an SNRI approved for depression in a number of countries outside of the United States, was effective for FM pain reduction in a 3-month clinical trial (**Figure 6.15**). Milnacipran also demonstrated durability of efficacy during a 6-month extension trial of patients

FIGURE 6.10 — Improvement in Average Pain Severity With Duloxetine

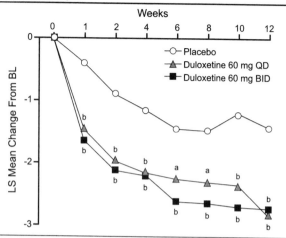

Phase 3 study: female patients (N=354).

[a] P <0.05.

[b] P ≤0.001 vs placebo.

Arnold LM, et al. *Pain*. 2005;119:5-15.

who were responders in the 12-week RCT (**Figure 6.16**).[10] The most common side effects were nausea, constipation, hyperhydrosis, and dizziness. However, milnacipran is currently not available in the United States.

Tricyclic Antidepressants

The first RCTs in FM utilized low doses of tricyclic antidepressants, most notably amitriptyline. Individual trials and meta-analyses have been favorable, with clinically significant improvement in 25% to 45% of patients (**Table 6.6**).[6,11,12] The doses of amitriptyline that have been studied were 25 to 50 mg, usually given as a single bedtime dose. For amitriptyline, there was a 4.2 odds ratio for efficacy compared with placebo (**Figure 6.17**).[13]

Cyclobenzaprine, although marketed as a muscle relaxant, is structurally a tricyclic, with similar efficacy and adverse side effects as amitriptyline. Cyclobenzaprine has been studied in FM RCTs with doses of 10 to 30 mg

FIGURE 6.11 — Improvement in Function (FIQ) With Duloxetine

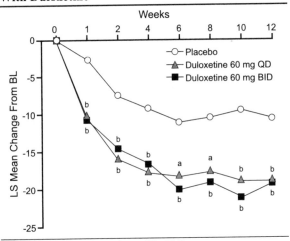

Phase 3 study: female patients (N=354).

a P <0.05.

b P ≤0.001 vs placebo.

Arnold LM, et al. *Pain*. 2005;119:5-15.

at bedtime (**Table 6.6**).[6] Even at these low doses, dry mouth, constipation, fluid retention, weight gain, grogginess, and difficulty concentrating are common with all the tricyclics. Such side effects and possible cardiotoxicity are especially problematic when using these medications in elderly patients. Tricyclic medications should be started at very low doses (eg, 5 to 10 mg) 1 to 3 hours before bedtime. The dose may be increased by 5 mg at 2-week intervals. The most consistently observed improvements noted with the tricyclics may have been attributable to the sedative effects. In many of the trials, comorbid psychiatric disorders were not evaluated and there was limited assessment of psychiatric or functional outcomes.

Selective Serotonin Reuptake Inhibitors

The next group of medications studied in FM were the selective serotonin reuptake inhibitors (SSRIs). In

FIGURE 6.12 — Pooled Data: Duloxetine Efficacy in Fibromyalgia Patients With and Without Major Depressive Disorder

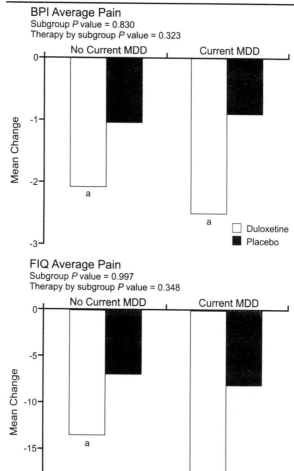

a P <0.001 vs placebo.
b P <0.01 vs placebo.

Arnold LM, et al. *J Womens Health*. 2007;16:1145-1158.

FIGURE 6.13 — Pooled Data: Treatment-Emergent Adverse Events Reported by >5% of Patients in the Duloxetine Group and Twice the Rate of Placebo

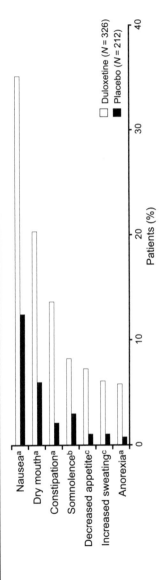

Arnold LM, et al. *J Womens Health*. 2007;16:1145-1156.

[a] $P \leq 0.001$ vs placebo.
[b] $P \leq 0.05$ vs placebo.
[c] $P \leq 0.01$ vs placebo.

FIGURE 6.14 — ≥50% Improvement in Average Pain Scores With Duloxetine in 3- and 6-Month Treatment Phases

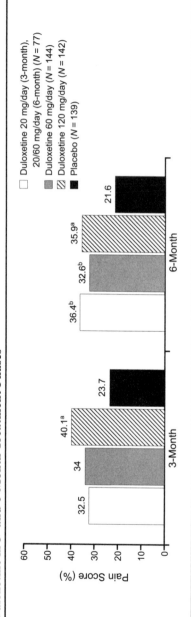

[a] P ≤0.01 vs placebo.
[b] P ≤0.05.

Russell IJ, et al. *Pain*. 2008;136(3):432-444.

FIGURE 6.15 — Efficacy of Milnacipran in Initial Fibromyalgia Randomized Clinical Trial

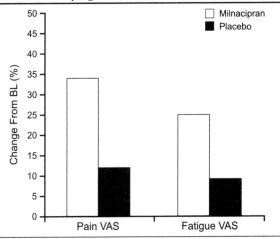

Gendreau RM, et al. *J Rheumatol.* 2005;32:1975-1985.

the first RCT, fluoxetine 20 mg/day was not superior to placebo.[14] However, fluoxetine 20 mg in the morning with amitriptyline 25 mg at bedtime was found to be effective (**Figure 6.18**).[15] Furthermore, the combination of both drugs was more effective than either alone. In a dose-escalation trial, 20 mg/day to a maximum of 80 mg/day of fluoxetine was more effective than placebo (**Figure 6.19**).[16] The mean dose was 40 mg/day. In these two trials with fluoxetine, the improvement of pain was independent of change in mood. Inconsistent results have been noted in small studies using fluvoxamine or citalopram in patients with FM.[6] However, a more recent study found paroxetine to be effective in FM.[6]

None of the SSRIs are FDA approved for the treatment of FM.

Other CNS-Active Medications

The short-acting nonbenzodiazepenes, including zolpidem and zopiclone, improved sleep in FM patients but did not improve pain (**Table 6.7**).[17,18] An RCT demonstrated efficacy with pramipexole, including pain, but

FIGURE 6.16 — Mean Change in Pain With Milnacipran

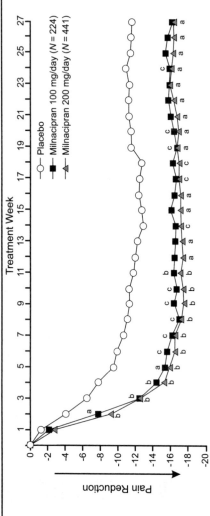

TABLE 6.6 — Tricyclics in Fibromyalgia

	Amitriptyline	Cyclobenzaprine
Placebo-controlled trials	• Goldenberg, 1985	• Quimby, 1989
	• Carette, 1986	• Carette, 1994
	• Carette, 1994	• Reynolds, 1991
Dose (mg)	25-50	10-40
Duration (weeks)	6-26	4-12
Efficacy	All showed modest efficacy	Two showed efficacy

Arnold LM, et al. *Psychosomatics.* 2000;41:104-113.

FIGURE 6.17 — Efficacy of Various Medications in Initial Fibromyalgia Trials

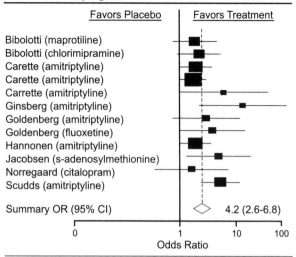

O'Malley PG, et al. *J Gen Intern Med.* 2000;15:659-666.

the use of other analgesics, including opioids, was permitted during that study.[19] Sodium oxybate (the sodium salt of gamma hydroxybutyrate), which has only been approved for the treatment of narcolepsy, was found to be more effective than placebo in pain, function, and global well-being.[20] A 5-HT$_3$ receptor antagonist, tropisetron, has been effective for pain relief in several short RCTs but the trials have been in one center and the drug is not currently available in the United States.[21] There are 5-HT$_3$ receptors present on both inhibitory dorsal horn interneurons and primary nociceptive afferents.

Analgesics, Anti-inflammatory Medications, and Others

There is no evidence that anti-inflammatory medications are efficacious as monotherapy in FM (**Table 6.8**). Prednisone 20 mg/day was no more effective than placebo in a short RCT.[22] Ibuprofen and naproxen were no better than placebo, although when combined with antidepres-

FIGURE 6.18 — Combination Treatment With Fluoxetine and Amitriptyline

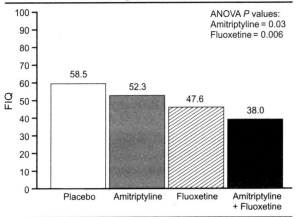

ANOVA *P* values:
Amitriptyline = 0.03
Fluoxetine = 0.006

Goldenberg D, et al. *Arthritis Rheum.* 1996;39:1852-1859.

FIGURE 6.19 — Fluoxetine in Fibromyalgia

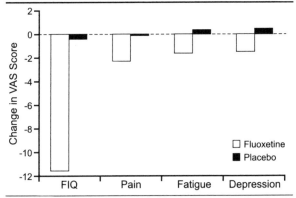

Dose 10 mg to 80 mg (45 mean). Fluoxetine vs placebo significant differences, $P=0.01$.

Arnold LM, et al. *Am J Med.* 2002;112:191-197.

sants, they may have had slight efficacy.[11,23] The NMDA-receptor antagonists, ketamine and dextromethorphan, have demonstrated mixed results.[24] Female FM patients treated with tramadol plus increasing concentrations of dextromethorphan seemed to have some additional pain

TABLE 6.7 — Sedatives and Hypnotics in Fibromyalgia

- Short-acting nonbenzodiazepine sedatives:
  - Zolpidem and zopiclone improved sleep in FM patients
  - Did not improve pain, not useful as monotherapy
  - No data on long-term use in FM
- Single study demonstrated efficacy with pramipexole, but other analgesics, including opioids, were permitted
- Gamma hydroxybutyrate/sodium oxybate (sodium salt of GHB) approved as orphan drug for narcolepsy:
  - Clinical data in FM show significant improvement vs placebo on composite of pain VAS, FIQ, patient global assessment; significant improvement in sleep quality
  - Distribution tightly restricted due to high abuse potential; may limit its applicability to FM
- A 5-HT$_3$ receptor antagonist, tropisetron, was effective in trials at one center

Drewes AM, et al. *Scand J Rheumatol.* 1991;20:288-293; Grönblad M, et al. *Clin Rheumatol.* 1993;12:186-191; Moldofsky H, et al. *J Rheumatol.* 1996;23:529-533; Scharf MB, et al. *J Rheumatol.* 2003;30:1070-1074; Holman AJ, Myers RR. *Arthritis Rheum.* 2005;52:2495-2505.

TABLE 6.8 — Anti-inflammatory Medications in Fibromyalgia

- Double-blind crossover trial showed that prednisone 20 mg/day was not better than placebo
- NSAIDs not effective in FM, although may have synergistic effect when combined with centrally-acting medications
- No evidence that FM is an immune or inflammatory disease

Goldenberg DL, et al. *Arthritis Rheum.* 1986;29:1371-1377; Clark S, et al. *J Rheumatol.* 1985;12:980-983.

relief with the dextromethorphan. Ketamine is impractical because of its parenteral administration and is viewed as an anesthetic.[25]

The only analgesic that has demonstrated efficacy in FM is tramadol.[26] In a randomized, double-blind, parallel group study of 315 patients, tramadol/acetaminophen 37.5-mg/325-mg tablets, 1 to 8/day with a mean of 4/day, was compared with placebo. The primary outcome measure, time to discontinue therapy, was significantly longer in the tramadol-treated group (**Figure 6.20**).

There are no RCTs of opioids in FM. Opiate use did not reduce pain intensity or pain symptoms in open-label studies in FM. There are experimental data which indicate that opioids may actually increase hyperalgesia in central pain states because of neuroadaptive changes enhancing nociceptive output. Their use in FM is controversial due to abuse potential and lack of efficacy data. However, a survey of US academic medical centers indicated opioid use in 14% of FM patients.

One novel pharmacologic approach in FM included growth hormone (GH), since subsets of FM patients have low serum GH levels.[27] This approach was modestly effective in a trial in which low GH levels in patients with FM were brought to normal with daily injections of GH. Sixty-eight percent of the GH-treated patients vs 26% of the placebo-treated patients experienced a "worthwhile improvement."[28] However, these results have not been reproduced in other centers.

REFERENCES

1. Goldenberg DL, Burckhardt C, Crofford L. Management of fibromyalgia syndrome. *JAMA*. 2004;292(19):2388-2395.

2. Crofford LJ, Rowbotham MC, Mease PJ, et al; Pregabalin 1008-105 Study Group. Pregabalin for the treatment of fibromyalgia syndrome: results of a randomized, double-blind, placebo-controlled trial. *Arthritis Rheum*. 2005;52(4):1264-1273.

3. Arnold LM, Russell IJ, Diri EW, et al. A 14-week, randomized, double-blinded, placebo-controlled monotherapy trial of pregabalin in patients with fibromyalgia. *J Pain*. 2008;9(9):792-805.

4. Crofford LJ, Mease PJ, Simpson SL, et al. Fibromyalgia relapse evaluation and efficacy for durability of meaningful relief (FREEDOM): a 6-month, double-blind, placebo-controlled trial with pregabalin. *Pain*. 2008;136(3):419-431.

5. Arnold LM, Goldenberg DL, Stanford SB, et al. Gabapentin in the treatment of fibromyalgia: a randomized, double-blind, placebo-controlled, multicenter trial. *Arthritis Rheum*. 2007;56(4):1336-1344.

6. Goldenberg DL. Pharmacological treatment of fibromyalgia and other chronic musculoskeletal pain. *Best Pract Res Clin Rheumatol*. 2007;21(3):499-511.

FIGURE 6.20 — Tramadol/Acetaminophen in Fibromyalgia

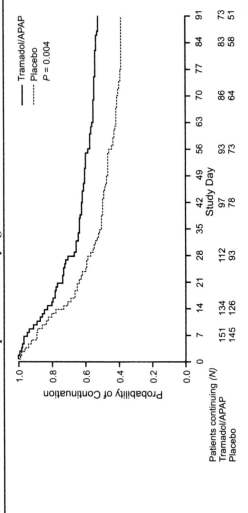

Bennett RM, et al. *Am J Med.* 2003;114:537-545.

7. Arnold LM, Lu Y, Crofford LJ, et al. A double-blind, multicenter trial comparing duloxetine with placebo in the treatment of fibromyalgia patients with or without major depressive disorder. *Arthritis Rheum.* 2004;50(9):2974-2984.

8. Abeles AM, Pillinger MH, Solitar BM, Abeles M. Narrative review: the pathophysiology of fibromyalgia. *Ann Intern Med.* 2007;146(10):726-734.

9. Russell IJ, Mease PJ, Smith TR, et al. Efficacy and safety of duloxetine for treatment of fibromyalgia in patients with or without major depressive disorder: results from a 6-month, randomized, double-blind, placebo-controlled, fix-dose trial. *Pain.* 2008;136(3):432-444.

10. Clauw DJ, Palmer RH, Vitton O, et al. The efficacy and safety of milnacipran in the treatment of fibromyalgia. *Arthritis Rheum.* 2007;56(suppl 9):S306. Abstract No. 716.

11. Goldenberg DL, Felson DT, Dinerman H. A randomized, controlled trial of amitriptyline and naproxen in the treatment of patients with fibromyalgia. *Arthritis Rheum.* 1986;29(11):1371-1377.

12. Arnold LM, Keck PE Jr, Welge JA. Antidepressant treatment of fibromyalgia. A meta-analysis and review. *Psychosomatics.* 2000;41(2):104-113.

13. O'Malley PG, Balden E, Tomkins G, Santoro J, Kroenke K, Jackson JL. Treatment of fibromyalgia with antidepressants: a meta-analysis. *J Gen Intern Med.* 2000;15(9):659-666.

14. Wolfe F, Cathey MA, Hawley DJ. A double-blind placebo controlled trial of fluoxetine in fibromyalgia. *Scand J Rheumatol.* 1994;23(5):255-259.

15. Goldenberg D, Mayskiy M, Mossey C, Ruthazer R, Schmid C. A randomized, double-blind crossover trial of fluoxetine and amitriptyline in the treatment of fibromyalgia. *Arthritis Rheum.* 1996;39(11):1852-1859.

16. Arnold LM, Hess EV, Hudson JI, Welge JA, Berno SE, Keck PE Jr. A randomized, placebo-controlled, double-blind, flexible-dose study of fluoxetine in the treatment of women with fibromyalgia. *Am J Med.* 2002;112(3):191-197.

17. Drewes AM, Andreasen A, Jennum P, Nielsen KD. Zopiclone in the treatment of sleep abnormalities in fibromyalgia. *Scand J Rheumatol.* 1991;20(4):288-293.

18. Gronblad M, Nykanen J, Konttinen Y, Jarvinen E, Helve T. Effect of zipoclone on sleep quality, morning stiffness, widespread tenderness and pain and general discomfort in primary fibromyalgia patients. A double-blind randomized trial. *Clin Rheumatol.* 1993;12(2):186-191.

6

19. Holman AJ, Myers RR. A randomized, double-blind, placebo-controlled trial of pramipexole, a dopamine agonist, in patients with fibromyalgia receiving concomitant medications. *Arthritis Rheum.* 2005;52(8):2495-2505.

20. Scharf MB, Baumann M, Berkowitz DV. The effects of sodium oxybate on clinical symptoms and sleep patterns in patients with fibromyalgia. *J Rheumatol.* 2003;30(5):1070-1074.

21. Haus U, Varga B, Stratz T, Späth M, Müller W. Oral treatment of fibromyalgia with tropisetron given over 28 days: influence on functional and vegetative symptoms, psychometric parameters and pain. *Scand J Rheumatol Suppl.* 2000;113:55-58.

22. Clark S, Tindall E, Bennett RM. A double blind crossover trial of prednisone versus placebo in the treatment of fibrositis. *J Rheumatol.* 1985;12(5):980-983.

23. Russell IJ, Fletcher EM, Michalek JE, McBroom PC, Hester GG. Treatment of primary fibrositis/fibromyalgia syndrome with ibuprofen and alprazolam. A double-blind, placebo-controlled study. *Arthritis Rheum.* 1991;34(5):552-560.

24. Staud R, Vierck CJ, Robinson ME, Price DD. Effects of the N-methyl-D-aspartate receptor antagonist dextromethorphan on temporal summation of pain are similar in fibromyalgia patients and normal control subjects. *J Pain.* 2005;6(5):323-332.

25. Graven-Nielsen T, Aspergren Kendall S, Henrikksson KG, et al. Ketamine reduces muscle pain, temporal summation, and referred pain in fibromyalgia patients. *Pain.* 2000;85(3):483-491.

26. Bennett RM, Kamin M, Karim R, Rosenthal N. Tramadol and acetaminophen combination tablets in the treatment of fibromyalgia pain: a double-blind, randomized, placebo-controlled study. *Am J Med.* 2003;114(7):537-545.

27. Bennett RM. Disordered growth hormone secretion in fibromyalgia: a review of recent findings and a hypothesized etiology. *Z Rheumatol.* 1998;57(suppl 2):72-76.

28. Bennett RM, Clark SC, Walczyk J. A randomized, double-blind, placebo-controlled study of growth hormone in the treatment of fibromyalgia. *Am J Med.* 1998;104(3):227-231.

7 Nonpharmacologic Management

The nonpharmacologic treatments that have been evaluated in FM patients include (**Table 7.1**):
- Exercise
- CBT, including group and individual
- Patient and family education
- Various types of injections
- Physical therapy and its offshoots
- Massage
- Acupuncture
- Chiropractic
- Others.

Exercise, CBT, and patient education have been the most efficacious in clinical trials (**Table 7.2**).

Exercise

There are a number of reasons to postulate how exercise could be helpful in the treatment of FM (**Table 7.3**). The pain in FM can increase with physical activity; hence, many people with FM are sedentary. Most investigators believe that chronic pain results in a spiral downward, with deconditioning making FM symptoms worse at rest or with minimal exertion. Exercise has been helpful in the treatment of other chronic pain disorders as well as in mood and sleep disorders.

Cardiovascular exercise has been shown to be helpful in a number of studies in FM.[1] A large meta-analysis of approximately 40 clinical trials demonstrated that exercise was associated with improved physical status, daily function, and FM symptoms.[2] Most of the trials regarding cardiovascular fitness training in FM utilized a treadmill or stationary bicycle and many of them involved other types of exercise. Only six of the trials were of moderate to high quality and were purely cardiovascular fitness in nature. Those trials demonstrated significant improve-

TABLE 7.1 — The Nonpharmacologic Approach to Fibromyalgia Treatment

- Exercise
- Cognitive behavioral therapy
- Patient education
- Injections
- Physical therapy
- Massage
- Acupuncture
- Chiropractic
- Other

ment in pain, tender points, function, and mood with aerobic training (**Figure 7.1**). There was also significant improvement in global well-being (**Figure 7.2**).

There have been only two high- or moderate-quality studies on strength training which demonstrated improvement in pain, tender points, and global well-being in FM patients (**Figure 7.3**).[2] For strength-training exercise, it is best to begin with low-impact exercises and to avoid eccentric muscle contractions. There has been less evidence that flexibility or stretching alone has been useful, although it may be helpful in some individuals. The studies have also demonstrated that women with FM gain the same physiologic benefits from exercise, including cardiovascular fitness and strength, as do healthy women.

There have also been a number of studies demonstrating efficacy of water exercise, such as water aerobics or deep water walking.[3] A recent study found that an 8-month aquatic program was cost-effective in patients with FM.[4]

In most patients, it is best to initiate exercise a few months after the start of drug therapy so the patient may be less symptomatic and better able to tolerate the exercise program (**Table 7.4**). However, patients who are less symptomatic or who do not want to immediately begin taking medications could be started quickly on an exercise program.

Any cardiovascular exercise should be initiated slowly and incrementally with a target goal of 30 to 40 minutes of aerobic cardiovascular fitness training 3 or 4 times weekly (**Table 7.4**). Moderate-intensity programs

TABLE 7.2 — Nonpharmacologic Strategies: Evidence of Efficacy

Strong Evidence
- Exercise:
  - Physical and psychological benefits
  - May increase aerobic performance and tender-point pain-pressure threshold and improve pain
  - Efficacy not maintained if exercise stops
- Cognitive behavioral therapy:
  - Improvements in pain, fatigue, mood, and physical function
  - Improvement often sustained for months
- Patient education/self-management:
  - Improves pain, sleep, fatigue, and quality of life
- Combination (multidisciplinary therapy)

Modest Evidence
- Strength training
- Acupuncture
- Hypnotherapy
- EMG biofeedback
- Balneotherapy (medicinal bathing)
- Transcranial electrical stimulation

Weak Evidence
- Chiropractic
- Manual and massage therapy
- Ultrasound

No Evidence
- Tender-point injections
- Flexibility exercise

Goldenberg DL, et al. *JAMA*. 2004;292:2388-2395; Williams DA, et al. *J Rheumatol*. 2002;29:1280-1286; Busch AJ, et al. *Cochrane Database Syst Rev*. 2002;(3):CD003786.

TABLE 7.3 — Exercise Rationale in Fibromyalgia

- The pain in FM can increase with physical activity; hence, many people with FM are sedentary
- Belief that there is a spiral downward with deconditioning, making FM symptoms worse at rest or with minimal exertion
- Exercise has been helpful in the treatment of other chronic pain disorders as well as in mood and sleep disorders

FIGURE 7.1 — Improvements With Aerobic Exercise vs Nonexercise Controls

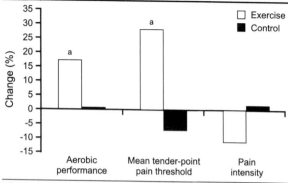

[a] Statistically significant.

Busch AJ, et al. *Cochrane Database Syst Rev*. 2002;(3):CD003786.

FIGURE 7.2 — Aerobic Exercise vs Untreated Controls: Mean Differences

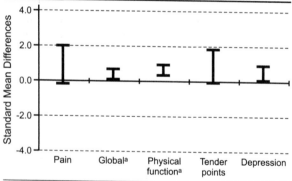

[a] Statistically significant vs untreated controls.

Busch AJ, et al. *Cochrane Database Syst Rev*. 2002;(3):CD003786.

(55% to 75% of age-adjusted maximal heart rate) are usually well tolerated but high-intensity (heart rate >150) aerobic exercise is poorly tolerated with high dropout rates. This was demonstrated in the clinical trials in which there were 13% to 44% attrition rates overall. However, compliance was much poorer in studies that used high

FIGURE 7.3 — Strengthening Exercise vs Controls: Mean Difference

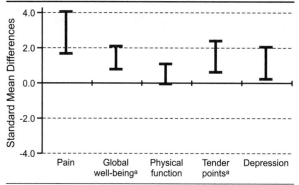

a Statistically significant vs untreated controls.

Busch AJ, et al. *Cochrane Database Syst Rev.* 2002;(3):CD003786.

TABLE 7.4 — Aerobic Exercise Guidelines in Fibromyalgia

- Begin 1 to 2 months after start of drug therapy
- Moderate aerobic exercise (60% to 75% of age-adjusted maximum heart rate [210 minus age] at least 3 to 4 times weekly)
- Exercise should be slowly and carefully introduced
- Strength and stretching should be incorporated gradually
- Start just below participant's total capacity; gradually increase duration to goal of 30 minutes of moderate-intensity aerobic exercise
- Both physician and patient should consider exercise as a "drug"

Modified from: Gowans SE, deHueck A. *Curr Opin Rheumatol.* 2004; 16:138-142.

intensity or unsupervised exercise. In general, it is best to start just below the participant's total capacity and gradually increase duration to goal of 30 to 45 minutes of moderate-intensity aerobic exercise.

Exercise should be prescribed in the same manner as a medication: explained in detail, with "dosage" written as a prescription. Since many physicians do not have the time or expertise for such discussions, referral to a physical therapist might be helpful. This is especially important in patients who are averse to begin an exercise program.

Cognitive Behavioral Therapy

CBT teaches patients skills to deal with illness more adaptively (**Table 7.5**). It can be provided individually or in groups by a variety of health care providers. It has been used effectively for the treatment of CFS, other chronic pain conditions, mood disorders, and sleep disorders. Many patients with FM view their illness as overwhelming. Due to the chronic nature of multiple symptoms, many FM patients feel helpless and hopeless. It is important to change this view into one in which patients feel some sense of control and power over their symptoms.

CBT allows patients to attribute feeling better to their own hard work and recognize that better health is due to their own efforts. They no longer feel helpless and passive, and can accept FM as a manageable illness. Typical components of CBT programs include (**Table 7.5**):

- Relaxation techniques
- Goal setting
- Problem solving
- Self-reinforcement
- Substituting maladaptive thoughts with positive ones.

There have been a number of studies demonstrating the efficacy of CBT in FM. In one study, 145 FM patients were recruited from a tertiary-care rheumatology clinic specializing in FM.[5] Seventy-six received six 1-hour CBT therapy sessions over a 4-week period along with their usual medical care, and 69 only continued their usual medical care. Physical functioning improved more in the CBT-treatment group, measured by improvement of >6.5 units on the weighted physical health summary scale of Short Form-36 (SF-36) (**Figure 7.4**). The efficacy of such a program compares favorably with the results of FM medication studies with drugs such as amitriptyline and fluoxetine. CBT and operant behavioral therapy improved pain and function more than attention placebo.[6]

TABLE 7.5 — Goals and Methods of Cognitive Behavioral Therapy

Goals
- Help patients view FM as a manageable illness
- Educate patients that through treatment they will learn skills to deal with symptoms more adaptively
- Realize that success is due to their own efforts
- Recognize that they are not helpless and passive
- Monitor thoughts, feelings, and behavior
- Anticipate problems and barriers, discover ways to deal with them

Methods
- Relaxation techniques
- Goal setting
- Problem solving
- Self-reinforcement
- Substituting maladaptive thoughts with positive cognitions

FIGURE 7.4 — Improvements With Cognitive Behavioral Therapy vs Standard Care Over 12 Months ($N=122$)

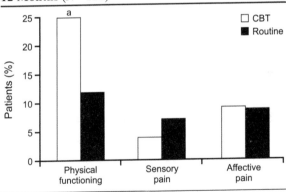

[a] Clinically significant; OR 2.9, $P < 0.05$.

Williams DA, et al. *J Rheumatol.* 2002;29:1280-1286.

Other Nonpharmacologic Options

Both exercise and CBT work best in combination with a formal education program. In one report, FM subjects were randomly assigned to CBT ($N=36$) or education ($N=35$) and both groups met for 90 minutes per week for 10 weeks.[7] Outcome measures, which were assessed pretreatment, posttreatment, and at 6 months, improved similarly in the CBT and education groups (**Figure 7.5**). Formal FM education, with a focus on self-management, improved the benefits of exercise, especially strength-training (**Figure 7.6**).[8]

There is also modest evidence for the efficacy of acupuncture, hypnotherapy, EMG biofeedback, balneo-therapy (medicinal bathing), and cranial electrical stimulation (**Figure 7.2**). Hypnotherapy and biofeedback have been helpful in some, but not all, reports in FM. There are conflicting reports on the efficacy of acupuncture in FM patients. Two trials found no significant difference between true and sham acupuncture[9,10] whereas other trials did report benefit from acupuncture. Sham acupunc-

FIGURE 7.5 — Cognitive Behavioral Therapy and Education in Fibromyalgia

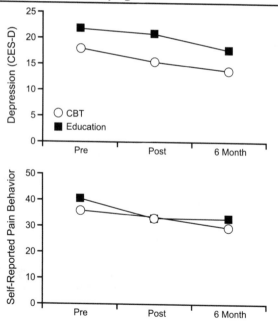

Continued

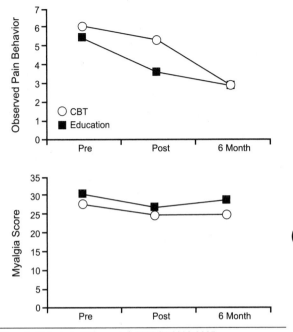

Nicassio PM, et al. *J Rheumatol.* 1997;24:2000-2007.

ture may have important therapeutic effects, making it difficult to evaluate overall efficacy.[10]

Meditation, relaxation, and stress management techniques were found to improve FM symptoms. However, historical or "waiting for enrollment" control FM patients were used for comparisons, since true blinding of such therapies is very difficult. Tai chi, Qigong, and yoga have demonstrated promise in the treatment of FM. However, only single studies have been done, and they were of low quality.

There is weak evidence for chiropractic, manual and massage therapy, electrotherapy, and ultrasound in FM (**Figure 7.2**). In one small, uncontrolled pilot study, chiropractic care improved FM patients' cervical and lumbar ranges of motion, straight-leg raising, and reported pain levels.[11] There has been only one small, controlled study of massage treatment, which showed that massage therapy reduced pain, reduced use of pain medications,

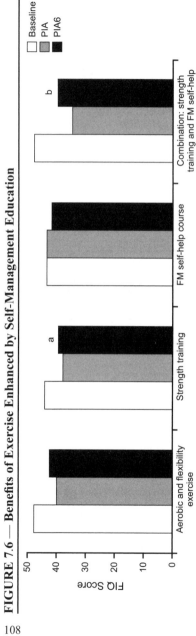

FIGURE 7.6 — Benefits of Exercise Enhanced by Self-Management Education

FIQ scores at baseline, PIA, and PIA6 in the four intervention groups.

[a] $P < 0.05$.
[b] $P < 0.001$ at 6 months vs baseline.

Rooks DS, et al. *Arch Intern Med.* 2007;167:2192-2200.

reduced impact of FM, and improved mood.[12] Although trigger point or tender-point injections with local anesthetics are often advocated, there have been no RCTs of these in FM.

A new innovative approach in both pain and depression involves neurostimulation of the brain. In one report, 32 FM patients were randomized to sham or real transcranial direct current stimulation (tDCS).[13] In this study, the anode was placed over the primary motor cortex or dorsolateral prefrontal cortex (sham area) and 2 mA of electrical stimulation for 20 minutes on 5 consecutive days was applied. The real anodal tDCS of the primary motor cortex resulted in greater improvement in pain as compared with sham or stimulation of dorsolateral prefrontal cortex. In another trial, transcranial magnetic stimulation (rTMS) or sham treatment was applied to the left primary motor cortex of 30 FM patients in 10 daily sessions.[14] The active rTMS reduced pain and improved aspects of quality of life more than sham treatment.

The recent recommendations from the European Union League Against Rheumatism (EULAR) regarding nonpharmacologic treatment included heated-pool treatment, with or without exercise, individually tailored exercise programs including aerobic exercise and strength training, and for certain patients, CBT (**Table 7.6**).[15] They also suggested that based on the specific needs of the patient, relaxation, rehabilitation, physiotherapy, psychological support, and other modalities may be indicated.

TABLE 7.6 — EULAR Conclusions Regarding Nonmedicinal Therapy for Fibromyalgia

- Nonpharmacologic treatments can play an important role in FM, including:
  - Heated-pool treatment, with or without exercise
  - Individually tailored exercise programs, including:
    - Aerobic exercise
    - Strength training
    - Cognitive behavioral therapy
- Need for more treatment centers that offer nonpharmacologic methods
- Further studies needed combining pharmacologic and nonpharmacologic treatment strategies for FM

Carville SF, et al. *Ann Rheum Dis.* 2008;67:536-541.

REFERENCES

1. Gowans SE, deHueck A. Effectiveness of exercise in management of fibromyalgia. *Curr Opin Rheumatol.* 2004;16(2):138-142.

2. Busch AJ, Barber KA, Overend TJ, Peloso PM, Schachter CL. Exercise for treating fibromyalgia syndrome. *Cochrane Database Syst Rev.* 2007;(4):CD003786.

3. Gusi N, Tomas-Carus P, Häkkinen A, Häkkinen K, Ortega-Alonso A. Exercise in waist-high warm water decreases pain and improves health-related quality of life and strength in the lower extremities in women with fibromyalgia. *Arthritis Rheum.* 2006;55(1):66-73.

4. Gusi N, Tomas-Carus P. Cost-utility of an 8-month aquatic training for women with fibromyalgia: a randomized controlled trial. *Arthritis Res Ther.* 2008;10(1):R24.

5. Williams DA. Psychological and behavioural therapies in fibromyalgia and related syndromes. *Best Pract Res Clin Rheumatol.* 2003;17(4):649-665.

6. Thieme K, Gromnica-Ihle E, Flor H. Effects of operator pain therapy in fibromyalgia syndrome (FMS). A controlled study over 12 months. *Z Rheumatol.* 1999;58:52.

7. Nicassio PM, Radojevic V, Weisman MH, et al. A comparison of behavioral and educational interventions for fibromyalgia. *J Rheumatol.* 1997;24(10):2000-2007.

8. Rooks DS, Gautam S, Romeling M, et al. Group exercise, education, and combination self-management in women with fibromyalgia: a randomized trial. *Arch Intern Med.* 2007;167(20):2192-2200.

9. Assefi NP, Sherman KJ, Jacobsen C, Goldberg J, Smith WR, Buchwald D. A randomized clinical trial of acupuncture compared with sham acupuncture in fibromyalgia. *Ann Intern Med.* 2005;143(1):10-19.

10. Harris RE, Tian X, Williams DA, et al. Treatment of fibromyalgia with formula acupuncture: investigation of needle placement, needle stimulation, and treatment frequency. *J Altern Complement Med.* 2005;11(4):663-671.

11. Blunt KL, Rajwani MH, Guerriero RC. The effectiveness of chiropractic management of fibromyalgia patients: a pilot study. *J Manipulative Physiol Ther.* 1997;20(6):389-399.

12. Brattberg G. Connective tissue massage in the treatment of fibromyalgia. *Eur J Pain.* 1999;3(3):235-244.

13. Fregni F, Gimenes R, Valle AC, et al. A randomized, sham-controlled, proof of principle study of transcranial direct current stimulation for the treatment of pain in fibromyalgia. *Arthritis Rheum.* 2006;54(12):3988-3998.

14. Passard A, Attal N, Benadhira R, et al. Effects of unilateral repetitive transcranial magnetic stimulation of the motor cortex on chronic widespread pain in fibromyalgia. *Brain*. 2007;130(Pt 10):2661-2670.

15. Carville SF, Arendt-Nielsen S, Bliddal H, et al; EULAR. EULAR evidence-based recommendations for the management of fibromyalgia syndrome. *Ann Rheum Dis*. 2008;67(4):536-541.

7

8 Comprehensive Management Plan

The optimal comprehensive management of FM must be tailored to the individual patient as well as to the health care setting. There is tremendous variability in the symptoms of each FM patient. Some patients will do very well with simple treatment that can be managed comfortably by the primary care provider. Other patients will require complicated pharmacologic and nonpharmacologic interventions and specialty management. Some of the FM management strategies utilized by primary care physicians will differ from those used by specialists (eg, rheumatologists or physiatrists). However, certain basic guidelines should be followed for the initial management of every FM patient (**Figure 8.1**).[1,2]

Accurate Diagnosis and Symptom Assessment

The initial management begins with an accurate diagnosis. This sounds simplistic but until recently, it took a patient an average of 5 years to receive a diagnosis of FM. That long period of uncertainty, doctor shopping, and costly testing can aggravate symptoms. Patients become distrustful of their health care providers or fearful that the diagnosis of some dreaded disease is being missed. A diagnosis, even if based on soft findings, is reassuring. An accurate diagnosis reassures patients that a progressive structural disease is not present and that they are not imagining their symptoms.

Once the diagnosis is made, the individual patient symptoms should be evaluated and their severity rated. Some patients will have much greater levels of depression, whereas others may be more troubled by cognitive disturbances. If comorbid illnesses (eg, OA or carpal tunnel syndrome) have been diagnosed, treatment of those should also be initiated.

FIGURE 8.1 — Initial Treatment of Fibromyalgia

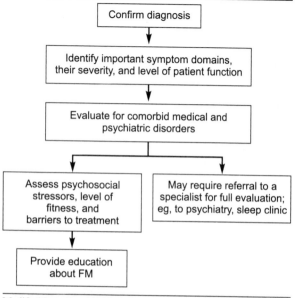

Modified from: Arnold LM. *Arthritis Res Ther*. 2006;8:212; Goldenberg DL. *JAMA*. 2004;292(19):2388-2395.

Optimal evaluation and management of coexisting mood disturbances are critical. Self-assessed depression is a risk factor for the development of FM, and high levels of depression and anxiety are associated with more physical symptoms, greater overall ill health, and more dissatisfaction with health in patients with FM. Although many clinicians evaluate mood informally using their gestalt, validated instruments are also available. The SF-36 and 12 Health Survey have been used in a number of FM studies.[3] If there is any question of a primary sleep disturbance, such as sleep apnea or periodic limb movements, referral should be made to a sleep laboratory and appropriate therapy initiated.

Some physicians have argued that the diagnosis of FM is typically disabling rather than enabling. They contend that the diagnosis medicalizes everyday symptoms and increases illness behavior. This only occurs if the diagnosis is not integrated with sound information and education about FM. However, it is important that the FM diagnosis not be linked to putative causes, such as an injury or exposure to an environmental toxin. In the overwhelming majority of cases, causal association of any chronic illness, whether it is FM or headaches, is speculative. Too often, such association leads to blame, inactivity, a sense of being victimized, and litigation. For example, in a series of FM patients, physical trauma was associated with receipt of disability compensation.[4] Trauma history was not related to pain severity or pain thresholds. In that study, the perception that physical trauma caused FM was a greater determinant of disability compensation than that for perceived emotional trauma, symptom severity, or functional disability (**Figure 8.2**).

Patient Education

Patient information should be provided in detail and, whenever possible, to both the patient and the

FIGURE 8.2 — Relationship of Trauma Onset of Fibromyalgia With Disability Application

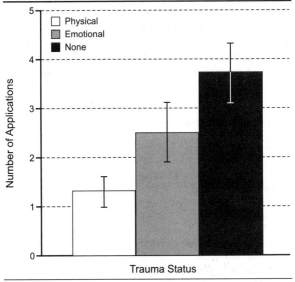

Aaron LA, et al. *Arthritis Rheum*. 1997;40:453-460.

immediate family (**Table 8.1**). It can be given in either the primary care or specialist setting. Patient education in the primary care office tends to be less formal and more conversational than in a specialist's practice.[5] Primary care physicians are faced with enormous challenges in caring for patients with chronic pain disorders such as FM. Our managed health care system insists that patient encounters be brief. Specialty referrals are often discouraged. There is little, if any, reimbursement for patient education. Therefore, optimal planning and use of precious office time and resources are important.

TABLE 8.1 — Patient and Family Education

- Primary care or specialist setting
- Core set of information should always be provided
- Pathophysiology best based on biopsychological illness model
- Anticipate common patient questions and concerns
- Recognize the wealth of patient misinformation
- Encourage patient participation

Often, FM education is best provided by specialists, working closely with a team of health care providers. This can be done in small or large group settings (**Table 8.2**). Rheumatologists or physiatrists are ideal specialists to develop such educational sessions, either as part of office practice or as a stand-alone education program. The patient's spouse and immediate family members should be encouraged to attend.

TABLE 8.2 — Structuring Group Fibromyalgia Education

- Generally, specialty clinic or office
- Schedule three to five FM patients together
- Utilize health care team
- Provide a detailed education session:
  - Group format
  - Standard didactic lecture
  - Open for questions, discussion
  - End with one-to-one advice
- Can be done in larger groups, such as a half- or full-day session

Part of the management plan should be to explain multidisciplinary therapy and to help the patient set up their individual plan (**Table 8.3**). Other physicians who can aid in managing the multidisciplinary therapy may include rehabilitation medicine physicians, psychiatrists, and pain specialists. Health care professionals who are often part of this team might include physical and occupational therapists, psychologists, and social workers.

TABLE 8.3 — Multidisciplinary Fibromyalgia Syndrome Treatment

- Physical medicine/rehabilitation:
  - Avoiding inactivity
  - Analgesic advice and nonpharmacologic treatment (trigger-point injections)
  - Cardiovascular fitness
  - Stretching, strengthening
  - Occupational therapy, work rehabilitation, ergonomics
- Mental health professional:
  - Psychopharmacology
  - Counseling
  - Cognitive behavioral therapy

A core set of information about the diagnosis, pathophysiology, and therapy for FM should be provided to all newly diagnosed patients. This should include the concept of functional illness, discussing the absence of organ pathology and the overlap with conditions such as CFS, IBS, and headache disorders. Focusing the pathophysiology on neural pain augmentation rather than muscle or joint pathology is important. The muscle pain and tender points can then be visualized as vulnerable anatomic sites that are hyperirritable rather than irreversibly damaged tissue. It is also then easier to explain the role of medications, such as antidepressants or antiseizure drugs, in influencing pain perception. Furthermore, the role of physical therapy, massage, tender-point injections, or acupuncture can be presented as useful in reducing muscle contraction and enhancing tissue oxygenation.

In this context, cardiovascular fitness and stretching make sense. Water exercise (especially in a warm-water pool), walking, and biking can be recommended. The role of alternative and complementary therapy should be discussed. Ninety percent of FM patients have used complementary therapies.[5] Although there are limited studies on complementary therapies in FM, three out of four FM patients will have tried herbs or lotions, 50% spiritual healing, 40% consulted with nontraditional health-care providers, and 30% tried dietary manipulations.[6] As discussed in Chapter 7, *Nonpharmacologic Management*, there is some evidence that acupuncture, meditation, and manual therapies can be helpful in some patients and should be mentioned. Patients should be encouraged to avoid alcohol, caffeine, and cigarettes, but cautioned about radical dietary changes or unproven nutritional supplements. This is also a good opportunity to discuss the many self-help books and overzealous claims for cure in a nonjudgmental fashion.

Patients should be encouraged to seek reliable sources of information; there are a number of excellent web sites, including those sponsored by the Arthritis Foundation, the American College of Rheumatology, the Fibromyalgia Network, and the Oregon FM web site.

The typical course of FM should be reviewed (**Table 8.4**). Patients need to be reassured that FM does not morph into another disease, such as SLE or multiple sclerosis. They should be reassured that there will be

TABLE 8.4 — Explaining the Typical Outcome in Fibromyalgia

- FM does not herald the onset of a systemic disease
- There is no progressive, structural, or organ damage
- Most patients seen in specialty practice have chronic, persistent symptoms
- Patients seen in a primary care setting more commonly report complete remission of symptoms
- Most patients continue to work, but 10% to 15% are disabled
- There is often adverse impact on work and leisure activities
- Quality of life for most patients improves with medical management

Granges G, et al. *J Rheumatol*. 1994;21:523-529; Felson DT, Goldenberg DL. *Arthritis Rheum*. 1986;29:1522-1526.

no permanent structural damage to their brain or body, implying reversibility of their symptoms.

Discussing outcome may vary also with the health care setting. In the primary care setting, FM more often remits spontaneously. For example, 2 years after the diagnosis of FM and with minimal intervention, 50% of community FM patients had a remission of their symptoms and were off all medications.[7] In our rheumatology clinic, we surveyed patients 14 years following their diagnosis of FM.[8] Two thirds of these patients felt better than when they were first diagnosed and 70% felt that their symptoms interfered little, if at all, with their daily activities or work. Only 9% had to leave their job because of FM. Nevertheless, most FM patients seen by rheumatologists or other specialists will have chronic pain and fatigue and will require long-term follow-up and management.

If the above educational guidelines are coupled with the FM diagnosis, patients typically report that the diagnosis was enabling, not disabling (**Figure 8**.3).[9,10]

Furthermore, the diagnosis of FM decreases office visits, diminishes the number of tests and medications ordered, and is highly cost-effective (**Figure 8**.4 and **Figure 8**.5).[10,11]

FIGURE 8.3 — **Fibromyalgia Diagnosis Improves Patient Satisfaction**

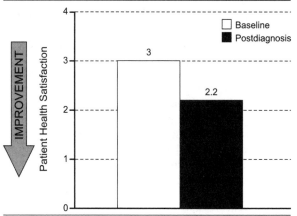

White KP, et al. *Arthritis Rheum.* 2002;47:260-265; Hughes G, et al. *Arthritis Rheum.* 2006;54:177-183.

FIGURE 8.4 — Positive Impact of Fibromyalgia Diagnosis in Clinical Practice

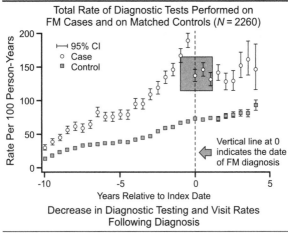

Total Rate of Diagnostic Tests Performed on FM Cases and on Matched Controls (*N* = 2260)

Decrease in Diagnostic Testing and Visit Rates Following Diagnosis

Hughes G, et al. *Arthritis Rheum*. 2006;54:177-183.

Medication Choices and Individualizing Therapy

The choice of initial medications should be tailored to the patient and follow current evidence-based guidelines (**Figure 8.6**).[1,2,12-14] Since pregabalin is the first FDA-approved drug for FM, many clinicians consider it to be the logical first choice for a patient with FM. Another approach might be to start a low-dose tricyclic at nighttime initially, especially in younger patients. In patients with some mild mood disturbances, an SNRI (eg, duloxetine) might be a good starting drug. Any of these medications should be initiated at low doses, such as 50 mg to 75 mg of pregabalin or 10 mg to 20 mg of amitriptyline at bedtime, or 20 mg to 30 mg of duloxetine in the morning. The dose can be gradually increased to recommended levels for FM over time, if tolerated.

Fibromyalgia patients typically complain of medication intolerance. Therefore, going slowly and anticipating potential adverse side effects are helpful. Simple analgesics, such as acetaminophen, may "take the edge off," although there is no evidence to that effect. However, if a comorbid condition (eg, OA) is present, nonsteroidal anti-inflammatory medications or other analgesics may be more effective. All patients should receive basic instruction in stress-management techniques and exercise.

For those patients not responding to initial therapy, referral to a specialist, such as a rheumatologist, psychiatrist, or physiatrist may help guide other therapies (**Figure 8.7**). The specialist needs to set aside a significant amount of time for the treatment and understanding of FM and related disorders. Physiatrists, as well as rheumatologists and neurologists, have the most experience in soft tissue injections. The role of standard physical therapy and techniques such as stretching, muscle strengthening, ultrasound, electrical stimulation, manipulation, acupuncture, and tender-point injections are often best reviewed by rehabilitation specialists. The importance of maintaining muscle flexibility and cardiovascular fitness is emphasized. The psychiatrist is especially critical in managing patients who may have major mood disturbances and require complicated psychopharmacologic regimens. They also should be adept at planning CBT or individual or group counseling. An anesthesiologist or another pain-management expert can also provide more knowledge regarding other analgesic techniques to consider.

In patients who continue to respond poorly to initial therapy, trials with combinations of drugs, such as an SSRI in the morning and a tricyclic at bedtime or an SNRI in the morning with pregabalin at bedtime, might be utilized (**Figure 8.7**). Adding tramadol or other analgesics may be considered. At this stage, a structured. progressive exercise and rehabilitation program should be considered. Patients with prominent psychosocial stressors or difficulty coping should be referred to a formal mental health program such as CBT.

In attempting to treat concurrent depression and FM, the dual reuptake inhibitors may be preferable to SSRIs (**Table 8.5**). With any of the antidepressants, the drug should be titrated to an adequate therapeutic dosage for an adequate duration of time to allow for response. If the patient does not respond to an adequate trial of that drug, a different class of antidepressants should be used.

Tests and Imaging

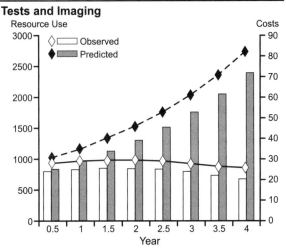

Referrals

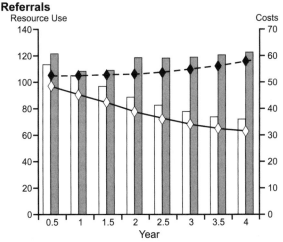

Continued

The combination of low or modest doses of an SSRI and a tricyclic drug should be considered in FM. However, it is important to be aware of drug interactions that may elevate tricyclic blood levels.

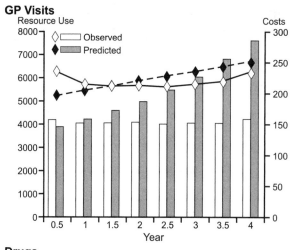

GP Visits

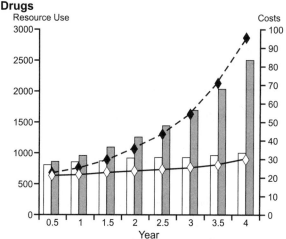

Drugs

Annemans L, et al. *Arthritis Rheum.* 2008;58:895-902.

A wide discrepancy exists in treatment preferences among medical disciplines, based on subjective, professional group-bound factors.[15] There has been a greater utilization of aerobic exercise and multidisciplinary therapy by rheumatologists and rehabilitation specialists during the past 7 years, but the use of recommended, evidence-based therapies is still very low, especially among generalists.

FIGURE 8.6 — Initial Medication and Nonpharmacologic Treatment of Fibromyalgia

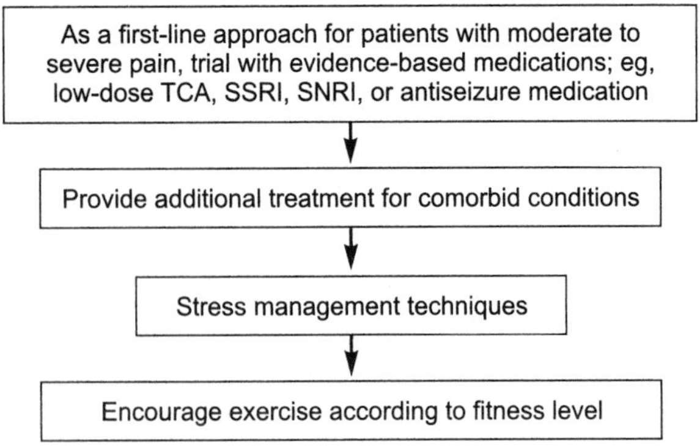

As a first-line approach for patients with moderate to severe pain, trial with evidence-based medications; eg, low-dose TCA, SSRI, SNRI, or antiseizure medication

↓

Provide additional treatment for comorbid conditions

↓

Stress management techniques

↓

Encourage exercise according to fitness level

Modified from: Arnold LM. *Arthritis Res Ther*. 2006;8:212; Goldenberg DL. *JAMA*. 2004;292(19):2388-2395.

FIGURE 8.7 — Further Medication and Nonpharmacologic Treatment of Fibromyalgia: Often With Specialists' Input

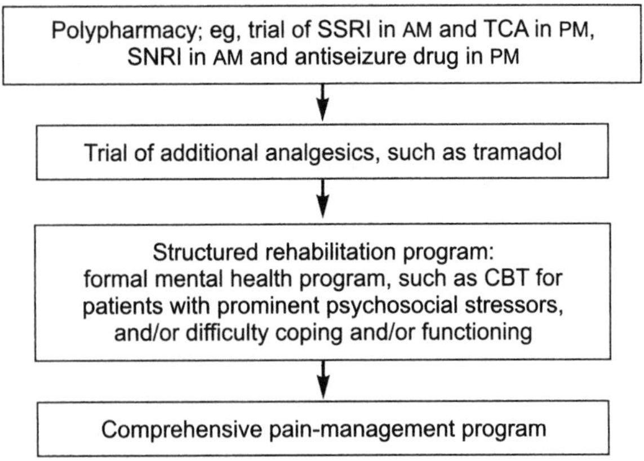

Polypharmacy; eg, trial of SSRI in AM and TCA in PM, SNRI in AM and antiseizure drug in PM

↓

Trial of additional analgesics, such as tramadol

↓

Structured rehabilitation program: formal mental health program, such as CBT for patients with prominent psychosocial stressors, and/or difficulty coping and/or functioning

↓

Comprehensive pain-management program

Modified from: Arnold LM. *Arthritis Res Ther*. 2006;8:212; Goldenberg DL. *JAMA*. 2004;292(19):2388-2395.

TABLE 8.5 — Strategies to Achieve Improvement in Comorbid Major Depression and Fibromyalgia

- SNRIs may be preferable to SSRIs
- Titrate to an adequate therapeutic dosage for an adequate duration to allow for response
- Switch to a different antidepressant if the patient does not respond to an adequate trial
- Consider a combination of an SSRI and a TCA (be aware of drug interactions with SSRIs that typically elevate TCA levels)

Whenever possible, treatment recommendations should be based on evidence from clinical trials. Although there have not been adequate trials to evaluate the combination of pharmacologic and nonpharmacologic management, experts believe that such integration is the key to optimal FM therapy (**Table 8.6** and **Table 8.7**).

8

TABLE 8.6 — Evidence-Based Management of Fibromyalgia

- Multidisciplinary therapy individualized to patient's symptoms and presentation is recommended
- A combination of nonpharmacologic and pharmacologic therapies may benefit most patients:
  - Nonpharmacologic:
    - Aerobic exercise
    - Cognitive behavioral therapy
    - Patient education
    - Strength training
    - Acupuncture[a]
    - Biofeedback[a]
    - Balneotherapy[a]
    - Hypnotherapy[a]
  - Pharmacologic:
    - Analgesic antiepileptics
    - Antidepressants
    - Analgesics, such as tramadol

[a] Treatment has limited efficacy.

Mease PJ, et al. *J Rheumatol*. 2005;32:2270-2277; Carville SF, et al. *Ann Rheum Dis*. 2008;67:536-541; Goldenberg DL, et al. *JAMA*. 2004;292:2388-2395; Clauw DJ, Crofford LJ. *Best Pract Res Clin Rheumatol*. 2003;17:685-701.

TABLE 8.7 — EULAR Recommendations for Management of Fibromyalgia

- Comprehensive evaluation of pain, function, and psychosocial context is needed to understand FM completely:
  - Because it is complex, heterogeneous condition involving abnormal pain processing and other secondary features
- Optimal treatment of FM mandates a multidisciplinary approach, including a combination of nonpharmacologic and pharmacologic interventions
- Treatment modalities should be specifically tailored based on patient description and presentation of pain and symptoms:
  - Reduction of clinical pain is optimized when all pain sources are addressed
  - Individualize treatment depending on pain symptoms:
    - Treat the pain
    - Address secondary conditions

Carville SF, et al. *Ann Rheum Dis*. 2008;67:536-541.

The recent recommendations from the European Union League Against Rheumatism (EULAR) focus on the importance of individualized therapy utilizing a multi-disciplinary team (**Table 8.7**).[12]

Attempts to identify FM patient subsets should help to individualize therapy. A study at the University of Michigan divided their FM patients into three groups based on psychological and pain profiles (**Table 8.8**). In the largest group, the patients had moderate control over pain, low levels of depression and anxiety with little catastrophizing, and were not severely tender. The second group of FM patients had no control over pain, very high levels of catastrophizing and mood disturbances, and were moderately tender. The third FM group demonstrated good control over pain, with little catastrophizing or mood disturbances, yet were the most tender. A patient from that third group might respond well to monotherapy with analgesic antiepileptic drugs. A patient in the second group would likely require intense multidisciplinary management, especially from mental health professionals.

In the future, classifying FM patients using psychological and pain profiles may be combined with biologic

TABLE 8.8 — Identifying Subgroups of Fibromyalgia Patients May Help Individualize Treatment

Group 1: Psychological Factors–Neutral (N = 50)
- Moderate control over pain
- Low depression/anxiety
- Not very tender
- Low catastrophizing

Group 2: Psychological Factors–Worsening Symptoms (N = 31)
- No control over pain
- Tender
- High depression/anxiety
- Very high catastrophizing

Group 3: Psychological Factors–Improving Symptoms (N = 16)
- High control over pain
- Extremely tender
- Low depression/anxiety
- Very low catastrophizing

Giesecke T, et al. *Arthritis Rheum*. 2003;48:2916-2922.

tests to provide more comprehensive predictors regarding response to various treatments. For example, brain imaging and baseline neuroendocrine studies have already demonstrated utility in predicting the onset of widespread pain after various stressors.

REFERENCES

1. Goldenberg DL, Burckhardt C, Crofford L. Management of fibromyalgia syndrome. *JAMA*. 2004;292(19):2388-2395.

2. Arnold LM. Biology and therapy of fibromyalgia. New therapies in fibromyalgia. *Arthritis Res Ther*. 2006;8(4):212.

3. Oswald J, Salemi S, Michel BA, Sprott H. Use of the Short-Form-36 Health Survey to detect a subgroup of fibromyalgia patients with psychological dysfunction. *Clin Rheumatol*. 2008 Apr 1. Epub ahead of print.

4. Aaron LA, Bradley LA, Alarcón GS, et al. Perceived physical and emotional trauma as precipitating events in fibromyalgia. Associations with health care seeking and disability status but not pain severity. *Arthritis Rheum*. 1997;40(3):453-460.

5. Goldenberg DL. Office management of fibromyalgia. *Rheum Dis Clin North Am*. 2002;28(2):437-446, xi.

6. Eisenberg D. Alternative medical therapies for rheumatologic disorders. *Arthritis Care Res*. 1996;9(1):1-4.

7. Granges G, Zilko P, Littlejohn GO. Fibromyalgia syndrome: assessment of the severity of the condition 2 years after diagnosis. *J Rheumatol*. 1994;21(3):523-529.

8. Felson DT, Goldenberg DL. The natural history of fibromyalgia. *Arthritis Rheum*. 1986;29(12):1522-1526.

9. White KP, Nielson WR, Harth M, Ostbye T, Speechley M. Does the label "fibromyalgia" alter health status, function, and health service utilization? A prospective, within-group comparison in a community cohort of adults with chronic widespread pain. *Arthritis Rheum*. 2002;47(3):260-265.

10. Hughes G, Martinez C, Myon E, Taïeb C, Wessely S. The impact of a diagnosis of fibromyalgia on health care resource use by primary care patients in the UK: an observational study based on clinical practice. *Arthritis Rheum*. 2006;54(1):177-183.

11. Annemans L, Wessely S, Spaepen E, et al. Health economic consequences related to the diagnosis of fibromyalgia syndrome. *Arthritis Rheum*. 2008;58(3):895-902.

12. Carville SF, Arendt-Nielsen S, Bliddal H, et al; EULAR. EULAR evidence-based recommendations for the management of fibromyalgia syndrome. *Ann Rheum Dis*. 2008;67(4):536-541.

13 Mease PJ, Clauw DJ, Arnold LM, et al. Fibromyalgia syndrome. *J Rheumatol*. 2005;32(11):2270-2277.

14. Clauw DJ, Crofford LJ. Chronic widespread pain and fibromyalgia: what we know, and what we need to know. *Best Pract Res Clin Rheumatol*. 2003;17(4):685-701.

15. Kroese ME, Schulpen GJ, Sonneveld HM, Vrijhoef HJ. Therapeutic approaches to fibromyalgia in the Netherlands: a comparison between 1998 and 2005. *J Eval Clin Pract*. 2008;14(2):321-325.

9

Controversies in the Management of Fibromyalgia

The Diagnosis of Fibromyalgia Is Not One of Exclusion

Because of the absence of any definitive physical findings, laboratory tests, or organ pathology, the diagnosis of FM is often considered only after every conceivable cause of pain and fatigue is excluded. This leads to long delays in appropriate therapy, unnecessary patient anxiety, excess costs, and inappropriate medical testing. The long delay in the diagnosis of FM can also adversely affect patient outcome. For example, in a 14-year follow-up of FM patients, those doing well had an average duration of symptoms of 14 months prior to the diagnosis of FM.[1] In contrast, those doing poorly had an average of 75 months of symptoms prior to the diagnosis of FM.

FM is not a diagnosis of exclusion any more than is the diagnosis of headaches. New onset of severe headaches may warrant an MRI in rare situations but almost never in chronic, recurrent headaches. Once a complete history and physical examination are unremarkable, there is little more testing that needs to be done in the diagnosis of FM. The initial work-up for a patient with probable FM is reviewed in Chapter 2, *Diagnosis and Differential Diagnosis*.

Is Fibromyalgia a Medical or a Psychiatric Illness?

Categorizing a chronic illness such as FM as either a mind disorder or a body disorder is harmful and unproductive (**Table 9.1**). FM patients often become defensive if they believe that a doctor is "telling me it's all in my head." There is evidence for both physical and psychological changes in patients with FM. It is fruitless to attempt to decipher which came first. Physicians should

TABLE 9.1 — Is Fibromyalgia a Medical or a Psychiatric Illness?

- Harmful and unproductive argument
- Fruitless quandary to work out what came first
- For all patients, symptoms are real and can be disabling
- Need a dual treatment approach targeting both physical and psychological symptoms

accept FM symptoms as real. Health care professionals do not question the reality of depression, headaches, or exhaustion. FM should be thought of in the same context. A biopsychological framework fits current concepts of FM and lends itself to a comprehensive, multidisciplinary treatment program.

Who Should Treat Patients With Fibromyalgia?

It is currently estimated that >50% of visits for FM are to primary care physicians (**Table 9.2**). Specialists are involved in about 25% of cases and 16% of FM visits are to rheumatologists. The ACR suggests that the role of rheumatologists should be primarily as consultants to primary care physicians. With an estimated 6 to 10 million FM patients in the United States, rheumatologists cannot accommodate such a large volume of FM patients.

The diagnosis and management of FM should be approached similarly to that of chronic headaches or chronic mood disturbances. These illnesses are largely diagnosed and treated by primary care physicians. Specialists should be consulted when the diagnosis is

TABLE 9.2 — Who Should Treat Fibromyalgia?

- More than 50% of visits are to primary care physicians
- Currently, 16% of FM visits are to rheumatologists
- The American College of Rheumatology suggests that rheumatologists serve as consultants (tertiary care)
- Other specialists should include:
  - Mental health professionals
  - Physiatrists
  - Pain-management experts

uncertain or when the initial management has been unsuccessful. Rheumatologists should advise the primary care physician with regard to team management, which often 'll include other specialists such as mental health pro-ᵃals, physiatrists, and pain-management experts.

Fibromyalgia Patients Thought cult to Treat?

ᵒtion relates to the uncertainty sur-
ᵃns are often skeptical when medi-
ᵉrified with objective data. We
ᵉxplanations to FM patients.
There are limited treatment options.

If a patient senses that their doctor or family does not believe them, which is a common complaint from FM patients, the patient may unconsciously exaggerate their illness or behavior. This may tie in with the increased prevalence of symptom reporting in FM patients and the overlap with somatization. Chronic pain causes stress, which may then cause individuals to function less well in their various roles. They may have difficulties with spouses, children, and work inside or outside of the home, which may exacerbate symptoms and lead to maladaptive illness behaviors. Such behaviors include social isolation, cessation of pleasurable activities, and reduction in physical activity and exercise. However, there is no evidence that malingering is any more common in those with FM than other chronic medical disorders.

The medical literature often paints FM as an intractable illness with very limited therapeutic options. Whether in the community or in specialty clinics, the notion that FM carries a poor prognosis is likely to create pessimism on the part of the patient and their health care providers.

Can Fibromyalgia Be a Cause of Disability?

Most FM patients followed in tertiary referral centers have chronic, persistent symptoms (**Table 9.3**). As noted earlier, in primary care practice, there has been evidence of spontaneous remission of FM in a significant propor-

TABLE 9.3 — Outcome and Disability in Fibromyalgia

- Most patients have chronic, persistent symptoms
- Most patients continue to work, but 10% to 15% are disabled
- Medicolegal issues are a disincentive to a patient's successful rehabilitation
- Work disability worsens the outcome in FM
- There is often adverse impact on work and leisure activities
- Duration of time without a diagnosis adversely affects outcome

tion of patients. Even in tertiary referral centers, most patients with FM continue to work. Depending on the outcome measures, 10% to 20% of patients with FM report that they are disabled. Even in those who have continued to work, there is often adverse impact on work and leisure activities from the FM symptoms.

There is significant evidence that disability status has a negative impact on outcome in studies of FM. It is very likely that medicolegal issues are a disincentive to a patient's successful rehabilitation. Once a person stops working, pain and function seldom improve and often worsen. The long-range outcome for patients with chronic pain, whether back pain or FM, is better when patients return to a productive existence. The medical profession must work with patients, claimants, insurance companies, and society to promote rehabilitation, self-care, and the ability of the patient to return to work. Therefore, an effective FM management program aims to maintain patients in the work environment.

Since the cause of FM is not known, any relationship to a precipitating factor should be reviewed by the physician on a case-by-case basis. Precipitating events may include physical trauma, emotional trauma, infection, surgery, and stress. The terms reactive and posttraumatic should be eliminated. The assessment of symptom severity and work capacity should include pain levels, functional ability, and psychosocial distress, using appropriate assessment tools.

How Can Health Care Professionals Improve the Care of Patients With Fibromyalgia?

The key to better care for patients with FM is better education about FM for both patients and physicians. It is important that the vagaries of FM be discussed with candor. Spontaneous remissions and exacerbations are the rule. Chronic symptoms usually persist and doctors must deal with comforting rather than curing FM patients. After all, as Robert Bennett said, "There is a universal human need for understanding bothersome symptoms in terms of a definitive diagnosis and plans for a cure."[2] FM clearly falls in that large group of human suffering that will never be completely understood or cured. Nevertheless, it can be effectively managed.

REFERENCES

1. Felson DT, Goldenberg DL. The natural history of fibromyalgia. *Arthritis Rheum.* 1986;29(12):1522-1526.

2. Bennett RM. Fibromyalgia and the facts. Sense or nonsense. *Rheum Dis Clin North Am.* 1993;19(1):45-59.

10

Abbreviations/Acronyms

5-HT	5-hydroxytryptamine
5-HT2A	5-hydroxytryptamine 2A
5-HT3	5-hydroxytryptamine 3
5-HTT	serotonin transporter [gene]
ACR	American College of Rheumatology
ACTH	adrenocorticotropic hormone
ALT	alanine transferase
ANA	antinuclear antibody
ANOVA	analysis of variance
APAP	acetaminophen
APS	average pain sensitivity
AVP	arginine vasopressin
BID	twice daily
BL	baseline
BPI	Brief Pain Inventory
BUN	blood urea nitrogen
BZD	benzodiazepine
Ca	calcium
CBC	complete blood count
CBT	cognitive behavioral therapy
CDC	Centers for Disease Control
CES-D	Center for Epidemiological Studies–Depression Score
CFS	chronic fatigue syndrome
CI	confidence interval
CNS	central nervous system
COMT	catechol-O-methyltransferase
CPK	creatinine phosphokinase
cps	cycles per second
Cr	creatinine
CRH	corticotropic-releasing hormone
CRP	C-reactive protein
CSF	cerebrospinal fluid
CWP	chronic widespread pain
DB	double-blind
EEG	electroencephalogram
EMG	electromyography

EP	end point
ESR	erythrocyte sedimentation rate
EULAR	European Union League Against Rheumatism
FDA	Food and Drug Administration
FIQ	Fibromyalgia Impact Questionnaire
FM	fibromyalgia
fMRI	functional magnetic resonance imaging
FMS	fibromyalgia syndrome
GABA	gamma-aminobutyric acid
GAD	generalized anxiety disorder
GH	growth hormone
GHB	gamma hydroxybutyrate
Glu	glutamate
GM	gray matter
GP	general practitioner
HPA	hypothalamic-pituitary-adrenal
HPS	high pain sensitivity
IBS	irritable bowel syndrome
IPL	inferior parietal lobule
LC	locus caeruleus
LPS	low pain sensitivity
LS	least-squares [pain score]
LTR	loss of therapeutic response
MCS	multiple chemical sensitivity
MDD	major depressive disorder
N	number [of subjects in study]
NCV	nerve conduction velocity
NE	norepinephrine
NMDA	N-methyl-D-aspartate
NMR	nuclear magnetic resonance
NREM	nonrapid eye movement [sleep]
NRS	Numeric Rating Scale
NSAID	nonsteroidal anti-inflammatory drug
OA	osteoarthritis
OCD	obsessive-compulsive disorder
OR	odds ratio
PBO	placebo
PCr	phosphocreatine
PET	positron emission tomography
PGIC	patient global impression of change
Pi	inorganic phosphate

PIA	postintervention assessment
PIA6	postintervention assessment, 6-month follow-up
PMR	polymyalgia rheumatica
PO_4	phosphorus
POMC	propiomelanocortin
PTSD	posttraumatic stress disorder
QD	every day
RA	rheumatoid arthritis
RCT	randomized clinical trial
rTMS	repetitive transcranial magnetic stimulation
SD	standard deviation
sec	second
SF-MPQ	Short-Form McGill Pain Questionnaire
SI	primary somatosensory cortex
SII	secondary somatosensory cortext
SLE	systemic lupus erythematosus
SNRI	serotonin-norepinephrine reuptake inhibitor
SP	substance P
SSRI	selective serotonin reuptake inhibitor
STG	superior temporal gyri
TCA	tricyclic antidepressant
tDCS	transcranial direct current stimulation
TMJ	temporomandibular joint
TMJD	temporomandibular joint disorder
TSH	thyroid-stimulating hormone
UA	urinalysis
US	United States
VAS	Visual Analog Scale
WM	white matter

10

INDEX

Note: page numbers in *italic* typeface indicate figures. Page numbers followed by a "t" indicate tables.

Abbreviations are for terms listed on pages 135-137.

11

11

11